P9-BZI-236

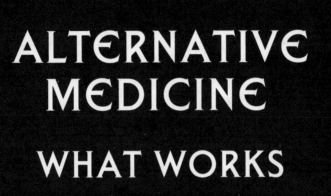

ALTERNATIVE MEDICINE

WHAT WORKS

A COMPREHENSIVE,
EASY-TO-READ REVIEW
OF THE
SCIENTIFIC EVIDENCE,
PRO AND CON

ADRIANE FUGH-BERMAN, MD

Editor: David Charles Retford
Managing Editor: Jennifer Eckhoff

Copyright © 1997 by Adriane Fugh-Berman MD. All rights reserved, including the right to reproduce or copy this book, or any portions of it, in
any manner whatever (except for excerpts in reviews).
Printed in the USA   First printing—March, 1996

Format and design © 1997
Williams & Wilkins
351 West Camden Street
Baltimore, Maryland 21201-2436 USA

Rose Tree Corporate Center
1400 North Providence Road
Building II, Suite 5025
Media, Pennsylvania 19063-2043 USA

Disclaimer

*This book's goal is to provide you with information that may be useful in
attaining optimal health. Nothing in it is meant as a prescription or as
medical advice. You should check with a physician or other healthcare
provider before implementing any changes in your lifestyle, especially if
you have physical problems or are taking medication of any kind.*

Trademark notice

*Because an important part of this book's purpose is to describe and com-
ment on various prescription drugs and other treatment modalities, many
such products are described by their tradenames. In most—if not all—
cases, these designations are claimed as legally protected trademarks by
the companies that make the products. It is not our intent to use any of
these names generically, and the reader is cautioned to investigate a
claimed trademark before using it for any purpose except to refer to the
product to which it is attached.*

CONTENTS

TO MY MOTHER,

ALINE FUGH BERMAN,

AND TO THE MEMORY OF MY FATHER,

DANIEL M. BERMAN

FOREWORD TO THE HEALTH CARE PRACTITIONER

Alternative Medicine: What Works is the right book at the right time for the many people who will read and use it. Read the author's introduction. Look at the numbers and the economics. Alternative Medicine is an idea whose time has come. Since the cultural conversation regarding healing is being advanced so rapidly on so many fronts, writing a foreword to this book affords an opportunity to take a look at a few of them.

As a primary care physician, I was happy to finally find under one cover an honest intellectual effort to present an easy-to-read discussion of alternative therapies from a physician whose credentials are just right. Many physicians are way down the road in their use of alternative approaches. Many others don't want to have anything to do with them. *Alternative Medicine: What Works* offers all readers an easy to use text with a scientific approach which should spur consideration of the use of alternative therapies in our practices.

Patients who read this book may be encouraged to come to us with questions about alternative therapies. Other patients who have not yet seen the book will continue to ask the questions they always have had about chiropractic, herbs, acupuncture and the rest. In both cases, our relationship with our patients and our ability to provide them with complete care will be enhanced by using this book as an aid to our discussions.

3

Acute care Western medicine is unmatched in saving lives, and in relieving immeasurable amounts of pain and suffering. The treatment of the chronic diseases, however, is where alternative therapies have found their place. There is a growing demand in our culture for a type of healing that flows from the "inside-out", that supports patient's efforts to reconnect mind, body, and spirit. Whether the departure from wellness is arthritis, obesity, depression, chronic pain, or others, there are legitimate approaches to alternative forms of healing that demand acknowledgment. By adding science and reason to the discussion, *Alternative Medicine: What Works* helps us to look for answers and feel safer in our choice.

Lewis M. Pincus, DO, practices internal medicine in Dallas, Texas. He is the creator and leader of To Life!, a lifestyle change workshop committed to the reconnection of mind, body, and spirit through science and inspiration. You will find him discussing wellness at http://www.columbia.net.

INTRODUCTION

In recent years, there's been an explosion of interest in alternative medical therapies. In 1990, when several medical researchers at Harvard conducted a telephone survey of 1539 English-speaking adults in the US, they found that one out of three had used some kind of alternative medical therapy in the past year.

Based on this sampling, the researchers calculated that Americans made 425 million visits to alternative practitioners in that year (vs. 388 million visits to primary care physicians) and that they spent almost fourteen *billion* dollars on alternative treatments—a figure that's certainly grown since then. [Eisenberg]*

(*Alternative* therapy simply means any approach to solving a health problem that's different from those used by conventional practitioners of Western medicine. It would be more accurate to call some of these therapies *complementary,* since they complement—rather than replace—conventional medical practice. But since *alternative* is the more common term in the US, that's the one I'll use in this book.)

Among patients with chronic diseases, the percentage of people seeking alternative treatments is even higher. In a survey of 184 HIV-positive patients in Philadelphia, 40% reported using alternative therapies. [Anderson] And in a study of 101 people caring for Alzheimer's patients in North Carolina, 55% reported trying at least one alternative therapy to

---

* All the studies cited in this book are listed by name (grouped by chapter) in the *References* section that begins on page 202.

improve their patients' memory, while 20% had tried three or more. [Coleman]

Alternative medicine is certainly popular. But does it *work*? That's the question this book set out to answer. Although there have been many books written on this subject, this is the first that reviews hundreds of scientific studies on dozens of treatment modalities.

If you're a layperson, don't let this talk of scientific studies scare you off. I've made every effort to write clearly and simply, and to explain things in everyday language. (Because some scientific terms are unavoidable, I've defined the most important ones in the next chapter, *Scientific terms explained.* You can also rely on the index, which is very thorough.)

As a consumer of health care, you can use this book in two ways: to identify the therapies you think might help your own maladies, and to convince physicians who treat you of the value of giving at least some alternative approaches a try.

If you're a health care professional, don't let this talk of simple, everyday language scare you off. *Simple* isn't the same as *sloppy,* and I've bent over backwards to be rigorous about the studies I've included and my interpretations of them. (For more on my methodology, see *A note to medical professionals,* which begins on page 17.) After reading this book, you'll be in a much better position to counsel patients about which alternative therapies are backed by solid evidence and which aren't. You may even decide to learn about some of these therapies yourself, and to incorporate them into your practice.

A final audience for this book is medical researchers. If that's your field, this book should give you lots of ideas for trials that need to be done—or done better.

Some kinds of alternative treatment—naturopathy, for example—aren't mentioned in this book because they combine a variety of treatments that are covered individually. But others—like reflexology—aren't mentioned simply because I couldn't find any good studies on them.

This doesn't mean they aren't valuable approaches—just that more scientific trials need to be run. So if you're a medical researcher, please get out there and give me more studies to cite.

SCIENTIFIC TERMS EXPLAINED

Some of the terms you'll come across repeatedly in this book may be unfamiliar to you. It's worth learning them, since they're universally used to explain the results of scientific experiments, and knowing them will not only help you read this book but will stand you in good stead when you read about scientific experiments elsewhere.

Fortunately, scientific terminology isn't hard to learn. That doesn't mean you're going to remember every single term after reading this chapter once. Just let whatever sticks in your mind stick, and ignore the rest. Then, when you encounter a term you're not sure about, refer back to this chapter, or look it up in the index. (I've boldfaced the terms where they're defined in this chapter, to make them easy to find.)

Study is a very broad term that covers almost everything that's looked at objectively. A human participant in a study—that is, one of the people whose responses, reactions or whatever are being studied—is called a **subject**.

A **case study** is a report on one unusual subject by a doctor. Both case studies and stories patients report themselves are called **anecdotal evidence**. Doctors joke that if we see two cases, we say we're seeing something "time after time," and if we see three cases, we call it a **case series**. Joking aside, a case series should consist of at least five cases. Case series are useful for indicating that something interesting is going on that may merit more formal study.

A **survey** is a kind of study that reports the results of interviewing people on whom no **intervention** is done. (Compare *trial,* below.) Since nothing new—no new drug, procedure, dietary restriction or whatever—is given to them or done to them, we say surveys are **observational**. Like the three studies cited in the *Introduction,* surveys simply try to discover how common a disease, treatment, condition or behavior is—or what **correlations**, or **associations**, there may be between various diseases, behaviors, etc. (There's a subtle distinction between a *correlation* and an *association* that isn't worth going into here.)

A **positive correlation** means that the more you have of A, the more you have of B. A **negative** (or **inverse**) **correlation** means that the more you have of A, the *less* you have of B. So, for example, there's a positive correlation between a high-fat diet and heart disease (the more fat you eat, the greater your chance of getting heart disease), and a negative correlation between eating broccoli and getting certain cancers (the more broccoli you eat, the smaller your chance of getting these cancers).

Correlations can't prove anything absolutely. For example, just because an increased number of storks in an area coincides with an increased number of births, that doesn't prove that storks bring babies.

How many people have a given condition at a given point in time is called its **prevalence** (for example, the number of color-blind people per 100,000 in the US today, or the number of people who were carrying tuberculosis bacteria on January 1, 1900). How many new cases of a condition occur over a given period of time is called its **incidence** (for example, the number of babies born in a given year who are color-blind, or the number of new TB cases in the last month). The study of prevalence and incidence falls into the field of **epidemiology**, which looks at patterns of disease and the factors that influence those patterns.

A **retrospective study** looks to the past for clues—you start with the disease and try to find out what caused it. For example, retrospective studies found that the prevalence of cigarette smoking among patients with lung cancer was higher than the prevalence of cigarette smoking among people without lung cancer. (Since you can't intervene in the past, all retrospective studies are observational.)

Retrospective studies can be large or small. To improve their quality, the **case-control** method is often used. This means that, when comparing a group with the disease to a group without it, the two groups are matched as closely as possible with regard to factors like age, sex, geographic location or any other variable that might affect the likelihood of getting the disease. The perfect case-control study would be of a group of identical twins where one twin in each pair developed a disease and the other twin in each pair didn't.

A **prospective study** is one in which subjects are followed forward in time instead of backward. Unlike retrospective studies, prospective studies can be either observational or interventional. Two famous prospective trials are the Nurses' Health Study, in which about 100,000 nurses have been answering annual questionnaires since 1976, and the Health Professionals Follow-up Study, in which about 50,000 physicians and other health professionals have been answering annual questionnaires since 1986.

By analyzing their responses, many associations have been discovered, including the positive correlation between hormone replacement therapy and breast cancer (that is, hormone replacement tends to increase one's risk of getting breast cancer) and the negative correlation between vitamin E intake and cardiovascular disease (that is, taking E tends to decrease heart disease risk).

Unlike a survey, a **trial** is a study in which the subjects receive an experimental intervention. Since you can only intervene in the present, not in the past, trials are always prospective. A **clinical trial** is one in which the subjects are human—as opposed to **preclinical trials** that use animals, bacteria, cells, etc.

In a **controlled trial**, at least two groups are compared. The **treated**, or **experimental** group receives the intervention, while the other—called the **control group**, or simply the **control**—doesn't. Or different groups may receive different interventions. The groups studied in a trial are also called **arms**.

In a **placebo-controlled** trial, an inactive pill or procedure—the **placebo**—is given to the control group. *Placebo* is Latin for *I will please [you]*; placebos got that name because any intervention, including simple attention, tends to make people feel better. Certain conditions, such as headaches, arthritis and hot flashes, are particularly responsive to placebos—as are some individuals.

Overall, the average **placebo effect** is an astonishing 33% (although it can range from much lower to much higher). In other words, an average of a third of the subjects in clinical trials will report significant improvement simply from being given a sugar pill (or some other placebo). So to demonstrate that a treatment works, you have to show that it does significantly better than the placebo that's given to the control group.

A **randomized** trial is one in which subjects are assigned to different groups as randomly as possible— by flipping a coin, or using a random number generator. If the researcher decides which subjects go into which group, or if the subjects assign themselves, intentional or unintentional **bias** can creep in and the groups may no longer be comparable (all the sicker patients might end up in one group, for example).

A **crossover** trial is one in which each patient is in each group at different times. For example, group A starts on drug X, and group B starts on the placebo; then, midway through the trial, the subjects are crossed over to the other arm (group A starts taking the placebo and group B starts taking the drug).

Blinding (sometimes, but less frequently, called **masking**) means that the researchers and/or the subjects don't know which group each subject is in. In a **single-blind** study, the subjects don't know but the researchers do (theoretically, it could also mean that the subjects know and the researchers don't, but there wouldn't be much point to that). Most nonsurgical studies are at least single-blind, since subjects' knowing whether they're getting an experimental treatment or a placebo is obviously likely to affect their responses.

In a **double-blind** study, neither the researchers nor the subjects know which group the subjects are in; all information is coded, and the code isn't broken until the end of the trial. (An exception is made when the difference between the two groups is so pronounced—everyone in the control group is dying, say, and everyone in the treated group is getting well—that it would be unethical to continue to deny the treatment to the controls.)

Double-blinding is important because researchers can give subtle, unconscious cues that can change subjects' responses quite independently of the treatment being tested. If the researchers don't know who's getting the treatment and who's getting the placebo, they can't put out those signals.

Saying that a treatment worked in 50% of the subjects tested obviously means a lot more if you're talking about 2000 subjects than if you're talking about two. So a good researcher involves statisticians before a trial begins in order to determine the **sample size** (the number of subjects) that will be necessary to show that the results are **statistically significant**—that is, unlikely to be due to chance.

Statistical significance isn't black and white; it's a matter of degree—what are the *odds* that this result was due to chance? It's measured by something called the **p value** (the *p* stands for *probability*). P values look like this: <.1, <.05, <.01, etc. *(< means less than)*. To translate a p value into English, move the decimal point two spaces to the right and say "percent."

A p value of <.01 means that the probability that the results occurred by chance is less than 1%. That's a good study. A p value of <.1 means that the probability that the results occurred by chance is less than 10%. That isn't so great, since it means that there's almost one chance in ten that the results are meaningless. In general, a p value of <.05 is considered statistically significant.

A large sample size helps to control for **confounding variables** (also called **confounding factors** or simply **confounders**). For example, a small trial on cardiovascular disease might happen to have a larger number of smokers in one group than the other. In this case, smoking would be a confounding variable, since it's known to cause cardiovascular disease.

If the sample size is large enough, however, one can assume that known—and unknown—confounders will be evenly distributed between the groups. To see why this is, imagine flipping a coin. If you flip it ten times, there's a reasonable chance it will come up heads 70% of the time (7 heads, 3 tails). If you flip it a thousand times, there's almost no chance it will come up heads 70% of the time (700 heads, 300 tails).

To put all this together—the gold standard for medical research is a prospective, randomized, double-blind, placebo-controlled trial with a sample size large enough to produce a p value of <.05 or lower. Many of the studies in this book don't achieve that standard— but then neither do most of the studies behind conventional medical therapies. If I limited the studies cited here to ones that meet that standard, this wouldn't be a book but an article...a short article.

Still, it's useful to know what the gold standard is, because everything—including trials of conventional medical therapies—should be held up to it. (Studies that don't meet the standard aren't necessarily wrong, but they're not proof. Future trials should adhere to the gold standard as much as possible.)

There are just a few more terms you should know. A **meta-analysis** is a relatively new kind of study in which you combine the results from a number of selected trials in order to come to some general conclusions. Meta-analyses are usually done when a number of small trials give ambiguous, conflicting or statistically insignificant results. When all of the decent trials are combined, there may be enough subjects in the combined treatment group to reach a statistically significant conclusion.

Let's say we're doing a survey of weights in a tiny village that has just eleven inhabitants. There are five children, who weigh 40, 50, 65, 65 and 65 lbs (the last three are triplets); three women, who weigh 105, 115 and 125 lbs; and three men, who weigh 150, 160 and 840 lbs (this last guy has a hormonal disorder).

If we add up all the weights, we get 1780 lbs; if we divide that by 11, we get 162 lbs. This is the **mean**—it's what we're talking about we use the word *average* in everyday speech. But it would be very misleading to say that the average person in this village weighs 162 lbs, since all but one of the inhabitants weigh less than that. To deal with situations like this, statisticians have come up with two other kinds of averages—the median and the mode.

The **median** is the value in the middle of the distribution—the one halfway between the bottom and the top. In this particular example, the median—105 lbs—gives a much better idea of the average weight than the mean does.

The **mode** is the value that occurs most frequently; in this example, it would be 65 lbs (the triplets). In some distributions, the mode is a better indication of what's representative than either the mean or the median.

The **FDA** (the Food and Drug Administration, a regulatory agency of the federal government) requires specific kinds of trials on human subjects before it will approve new drugs. (Animal studies and the like have typically been done before these trials take place.) A **Phase I** trial simply tests for safety; it's usually done on healthy volunteers, without a control group.

In a **Phase II** trial, the drug is given to people with the condition or disease to be treated; it supplies some preliminary data on whether the treatment works, and supplements the safety data of the Phase I trial. Phase II trials may or may not use a control group.

A **Phase III** trial assesses efficacy, safety and dosage, compared with standard treatments or a placebo. Phase III trials are usually randomized and controlled.

Phase I, II, and III trials are usually performed as part of an **IND** (an *investigational new drug* application to the FDA). After the Phase III trial is completed, the manufacturer can submit an **NDA** (a *new drug application*) which requests permission to market the drug.

Not routinely required, **Phase IV** studies are done after drugs are approved by the FDA and can be sold to the public. They're randomized trials or surveys that attempt to evaluate long-term benefits and risks.

Finally, **in vitro** (literally, "in glass") refers to studies done in artificial environments like test tubes, and **in vivo** to studies done in living organisms.

A NOTE TO
MEDICAL PROFESSIONALS

This book is intended to spark a reasonable discussion about alternative medicine, by surveying the scientific studies that have been done of it. Since I didn't have room to cover absolutely every alternative therapy, I've eliminated ones that aren't widely practiced, and ones on which few (or no) studies are available in English.

This latter reason isn't ethnocentrism, but rather lack of translation resources. It's true that translated abstracts are often available, but abstracts of studies in English so seldom accurately reflect the studies they purport to summarize that I had little faith that translated abstracts would be any better.

The studies I do cite in this book have been selected according to where they were published (the vast majority are from peer-reviewed publications), whether I believe they're reasonable, and whether or not they appealed to my own idiosyncratic taste. I've read them all, and have avoided secondary sources like the plague.

I've also made a point of choosing studies that are *accessible*. My pet peeve is running across an interesting tidbit in a book and flipping eagerly to the reference, only to find that it was someone's thesis, self-published, published in some unknown organization's newsletter, an ancient abstract presented at an obscure conference, or isn't available in English. Almost every study cited in this book should be easily obtainable at a medical library.

While this book should answer those who say there's no scientific evidence that supports alternative medicine, I'm well aware that evidence isn't proof. Just keep in mind that the converse is also true: lack of evidence doesn't equal disproof. Indeed, my clinical experience has taught me that alternative therapies are effective for a number of conditions for which I could find no published studies.

Few of the studies in this book are definitive. I've culled out the worst, but some downright mediocre studies remain, either because it was them or nothing, or because they may hold clues to promising areas for further research. Often, the mere fact that they were done at all is remarkable, considering the dearth of public and private support for alternative medicine trials. (As is well known, pharmaceutical manufacturers are loath to fund research on therapies that aren't patentable.)

Fortunately, times are changing, and so is the funding situation. Private foundations are interested in alternative therapies, the Office of Alternative Medicine at NIH has funded many projects, and alternative medicine research centers are thriving at Harvard, Columbia and the University of Maryland.

Medical education is also changing. Since 1973, Montefiore Hospital in New York City has had a residency program in social medicine that includes the study of alternative therapies. A fellowship in alternative medicine will soon be established at the University of Arizona, and numerous medical schools offer electives on the subject.

Because alternative therapies are often so cost-effective, third-party payers are even coming around. Chiropractic is covered by 85% of insurance companies as well as by Medicare, and many carriers also cover massage therapy or acupuncture, when they're prescribed by a physician.

It behooves us as practitioners to be familiar with therapies our patients are using. The studies cited in this book should make you feel more comfortable referring your patients to skilled practitioners of at least some alternative modalities.

As I suggested in the introduction, you may even want to incorporate an idea or two into your practice, or do research yourself into some area that needs further study. At the very least, I hope this book will open up a sympathetic discussion of alternative medicine, by convincing you that it's not all voodoo and witchcraft.

ACUPUNCTURE

Acupuncture is the insertion of hair-thin needles into specific points on the body to prevent or treat illness. It's one component of *traditional Chinese medicine* (or *TCM)*, an integrated system that's been used in China for more than 2000 years.

Most TCM practitioners also use herbal mixtures. Herbs—sometimes mixed with minerals and animal products (including cicada shells and cow gallstones)— are blended together in recipes that can be quite complex. Among the Chinese physicians who only use one therapy or the other, herbalists outnumber acupuncturists. (For more about the herbal component of TCM, see the chapter on herbs.)

According to TCM, acupuncture works by correcting the balance of energy, or *qi,* in the body. Qi (pronounced *chee* in Chinese and *kee* in Japanese) flows through 59 *meridians* that wend their way through the body. (No one has yet discovered anatomical correlates for these channels of energy, but the fact that they exist is made clear by the effects acupuncture can have on them.)

The movement of qi in the meridians can become deficient, excessive, stagnant or wayward, and any of these conditions can be influenced by inserting needles into *points* along the meridians. In classical theory, there are about 365 acupuncture points, but over time, the number of points has increased to about 2000. This is partly due to the development of localized versions of acupuncture that use just the ear or the hand, but the perceived superiority of complexity may have also contributed to the increase.

Which points are selected is important, but so is the angle and depth of the needle insertion; in fact, differences in these factors may cause opposite effects at the same point. *Acupressure* (pressing on acupuncture points with the fingers) can be substituted for needles, as can electrical stimulation of the points, or placing smoldering cones of the herb *moxa (Artemisia vulgaris,* or *mugwort)* on them. Needles are sometimes twirled to maximize their effect.

The most common side effect of acupuncture is relaxation and an increased sense of well-being. Adverse side effects can occur, but they're rare. In the United States, only ten incidents of injury to internal organs have been reported since 1965. Although acupuncture is widely practiced in China and Japan, only the same number of internal injuries—ten—have been reported since 1972. [NCCA]

A more serious problem stems from the use of reusable needles. Inadequate sterilization procedures have resulted in infections, including HIV and hepatitis. (One sloppy acupuncturist was responsible for 35 cases of hepatitis.) To avoid this problem, disposable needles are typically used today. [Kent]

Acupuncture was recognized in Western medical texts more than a hundred years ago. The 1901 edition of *Gray's Anatomy* states that "the sciatic nerve…has been acupunctured for the relief of sciatica," and Sir William Osler's *Principles and Practice of Medicine,* first published in 1892, recommended acupuncture for both sciatica and lumbago. [Lytle] (Osler died in 1919, and about thirty years later, in a bit of postmortem politics, the references to acupuncture were expunged from the seventeenth edition of his classic book.)

After the victory of the Chinese Revolution in 1949, there was a large push towards modernization. Some leaders proposed replacing TCM with modern Western medicine, while others supported tradition. To settle the question, many studies were conducted in the 1950s. Since these studies found TCM to be effective for many conditions, in 1958 the Chinese government decided to give it equal status with Western medicine. Today, physicians in China usually learn both systems.

Although acupuncture has always been practiced within Asian communities in the United States, general interest in it grew after 1972, when a *New York Times* correspondent had an emergency operation in China and was treated with acupuncture for a complication following surgery. Acupuncture schools have proliferated in the United States and other countries, and there are many variations of the practice, some of which have only the most distant relationship to Chinese acupuncture.

Soon after taking a job as medical director of an alternative medicine clinic, I received my first acupuncture treatment and was describing it to one of the staff. Another staff person interrupted me. Her voice dripping with scorn, she said, "You've never received acupuncture and you consider yourself Chinese?" Ignoring the implication that one's genetic heritage is optional, I explained that my Chinese mother told me never to trust an acupuncturist whose family hadn't been doing it for at least seven generations. While my mother may have a higher standard than most, quality and consistency are important traits for an acupuncturist.

The Food and Drug Administration (FDA) is finally considering taking acupuncture needles off of investigational status, where they've languished for years. This would open the way for acupuncture to be covered by Medicare, Medicaid and private insurance.

That's good news, because acupuncture is effective for a variety of conditions, and it can be used in situations where Western medicine has limitations (stroke rehabilitation, for example, or treatment of addictions) or where Western medicine would be dangerous (to anesthetize someone who can't tolerate normal anesthetic drugs, for example). There's a great deal of potential for the incorporation of acupuncture into our medical care system.

Thousands of studies of acupuncture have been done, but many of them have been badly described, uncontrolled, too small or otherwise inadequate. There have been problems with choosing appropriate placebo controls, and particular difficulties with blinding.

For example, if the only reason acupuncture works is because the irritation of having needles stuck into you distracts you from the pain you came in with, then the placebo should involve the same level of irritation, a requirement that taking a pill obviously doesn't meet. In several trials, acupuncturists pretended to needle the control patients (by pressing the tubes the needles come in onto the skin), but patients generally know whether needles are inserted or not.

Double-blinding is even harder to achieve. Needles can be inserted at points inappropriate to the diagnosis, but that can't be *double*-blind, since the acupuncturist will of course know whether the points used are real or sham.

One ingenious trial was blinded by having one acupuncturist evaluate the patient and another acupuncturist, who knew nothing about the patient, place the needles where the first acupuncturist instructed. In some patients, the points used matched the diagnosis; in other patients, they didn't.

Yet another way to try to control a study is to insert needles into nonacupuncture points. Some acupuncturists hold that since qi flows everywhere in the body, it's unethical to do this; the qi might be affected in unexpected or adverse ways. The same criticism applies to using inappropriate points.

The trials that use sham acupuncture (wrong or nonexistent points) often show that it has some effect—in some cases, as strong an effect as real acupuncture. Needless to say, this is extremely disturbing to those in the field. They spend years learning point location, and are understandably quite upset with the idea that stabbing patients randomly may be almost as effective as using real acupuncture points.

One final complication is that a study of acupuncture can only be as good as the person(s) choosing the points. There's a wide range of acupuncture training, and in practice acupuncturists develop their own idiosyncratic styles. If you ask ten acupuncturists what are appropriate points for a given condition, you might get ten different responses.

A minority of studies gave acupuncturists free reign to choose the points, to control the number of visits, and to use electrical stimulation if they wanted. Most studies, however, use formula acupuncture—that is, one acupuncturist chooses the points to be used. If such a study doesn't get a positive result, it may only mean that this sole acupuncturist chose the wrong points—or that acupuncture only works when it's individualized.

The scientific literature on acupuncture (in English) is quite sparse, and many ailments that are commonly—and, in my experience, successfully—treated with acupuncture have not been well-studied. More controlled trials should be done on pain and addiction, inflammatory bowel disease, depression, infertility and neurological diseases, among others.

Keeping all the limitations of acupuncture research in mind, here are some of the better studies:

Pain

In China, acupuncture is used for a wide variety of medical conditions, but in the United States it's accepted by conventional doctors—if at all—solely for the treatment of pain. Many chronic pain patients seem to be helped by acupuncture. This is fortunate, since several common prescription and nonprescription painkillers—aspirin, ibuprofen, naproxen and indomethacin, for example—can cause liver and kidney problems, ulcers and gastrointestinal bleeding.

One randomized, controlled trial, which even the American Medical Association thought was well-designed, followed 50 patients with chronic low-back pain. The patients were divided into two groups—one received acupuncture right away and the other was scheduled to receive it later.

83% of the immediate-treatment patients improved, reducing their average pain scores by half, while in the delayed-treatment group, a third got better and a quarter got worse. When the delayed-treatment group received acupuncture, 75% of them also improved. Forty weeks later, 58% of the patients who had received acupuncture (in either group) continued to show improvement. Ten patients who either dropped out of the study or received inadequate treatment didn't improve at all. [Coan 1]

In another study of 30 patients with neck pain, half received acupuncture and the other half didn't. 80% of the treated patients showed improvement three months later, with a 40% reduction in pain, a 68% reduction in hours of pain a day and 32% improvement in activity level. In the control group, 60% of the patients got worse and just 13% improved. [Coan 2]

With headache pain, acupuncture has shown mixed results. For example, it doesn't seem to work for tension headaches. Several studies comparing real to sham acupuncture found little difference between the two (both treatments helped). [Tavola, Vincent 2] Another study that compared acupuncture to physiotherapy (exercise, massage, relaxation, etc.) found acupuncture to be less effective. [Carlsson]

On the other hand, acupuncture sometimes seems to work for migraines. In a trial that compared real acupuncture to sham acupuncture in 30 patients with chronic migraine, real acupuncture was much more effective in reducing pain and medication use, and these effects persisted for at least a year. [Vincent 1]

However, in another study of migraine patients that compared acupuncture to a TENS (electrical stimulation for pain) device that was deactivated, no statistically significant difference was found. [Dowson] (In another study of 62 people suffering from chronic nerve pain after a shingles attack, acupuncture also fared no better than a mock TENS machine.) [Lewith]

In an uncontrolled Scandinavian study of 29 patients awaiting knee replacement for arthritis, acupuncture provided significant improvement in pain and range of motion, and significantly less use of painkillers; seven patients felt so much better that they decided not to have the surgery after all. [Christensen 1] But in an earlier sham-vs.-real acupuncture trial of 40 arthritis sufferers, both groups improved about equally. [Gaw]

In a small study on the effect of acupuncture on post-surgical pain, 20 patients underwent gynecological surgery and were then hooked up to intravenous pumps that administered painkiller when the patients pushed a button. Half of the patients received electroacupuncture while still under anesthesia; after they woke up, they used only half as much painkiller as the control group. [Christensen 3]

In a study of 90 patients who had a tube put down their throats into their stomachs (to diagnose or treat stomach problems), the half who received real acupuncture experienced less difficulty with the tube, less pain and less nausea than the half who received sham acupuncture. [Cahn]

For kidney-stone pain, acupuncture was found to be as effective as drug treatment. And almost half the subjects receiving drugs had side effects, while no one receiving acupuncture did. [Lee]

A study of menstrual cramps compared four groups. Group A received real acupuncture (at fixed, classical acupuncture points, with no individual variation), group B received sham acupuncture, group C received only extra office visits and group D received no intervention at all. In group A, 91% were able to halve a monthly pain score. 36% of group B improved, and 18% of group C. In group D, only 10% improved. During the nine months following treatment, group A used 41% less painkiller medication, while those in the other groups either increased their medication or stayed on the same dose. [Helms]

In a trial of chronic angina sufferers (patients who, despite intensive medical treatment, still had at least five angina attacks a week), 21 subjects received acupuncture for four weeks and a placebo pill for four weeks. Acupuncture reduced the number and severity of the attacks, and improved EKG readings during exercise. [Richter] However, another angina study found that both real and sham acupuncture reduced the incidence of angina attacks, so it's not clear acupuncture is effective for this condition. [Ballegaard]

One meta-analysis that looked at fourteen controlled trials of acupuncture for chronic pain found that the results favored acupuncture, although there were some blinding problems that could have introduced bias. [Patel] Another meta-analysis looked at 51 controlled trials and found highly contradictory results: the authors concluded that the efficacy of acupuncture for pain is not proven in the medical literature. [ter Riet]

Pain is notoriously difficult to study, and individual patients may experience relief even if formal trials are unimpressive. From my own clinical experience, I have no doubt that acupuncture is very helpful for many chronic pain patients.

Still, it's curious that the studies aren't more compelling—especially since acupuncture is more accepted in this country, and more likely to be covered by insurance, when used to treat pain than when used for other conditions. Physicians who pooh-pooh the idea of using acupuncture for other problems believe in using it for pain.

Perhaps this is because research has shown that the painkilling effect of acupuncture seems to be connected to *endorphins* (natural, narcotic-like substances produced by our brains). Conventional Western doctors have trouble with the concept of energy traversing invisible channels, but endorphins are something they understand. It's known that trauma can increase these natural opiates, and one argument used to dispute the effectiveness of acupuncture holds that it works merely by the counterirritant effect (that is, the pain of the needles takes your mind off whatever problem you're being treated for).

It's a silly argument, for a couple of reasons: acupuncture needles don't hurt much (unless you've really annoyed your acupuncturist), and acupuncture effectively treats many other problems besides pain. Endorphins can't begin to explain all of its effects.

Nausea and vomiting

Perhaps the clearest evidence of acupuncture's effectiveness relates to nausea and vomiting. Acupressure or acupuncture at the P-6—or Neiguan—point (it's about three fingerbreadths above the wrist) has been shown to be very effective in treating this problem.

A Chinese sailing enthusiast who suffered from seasickness found that he could control it by acupressure on the P-6 point; unfortunately, this left him with only one free hand for sailing, a perilous proposition. So he invented Seabands, elastic strips you wear around your wrists that contain a button that presses the P-6 point.

Seabands have been tested in a number of trials. In twelve of sixteen patients with morning sickness, they improved symptoms, compared to a placebo band that pressed on a nonacupuncture point. (Morning sickness can be difficult to treat because so many drugs are prohibited for pregnant women.) [Hyde] In a larger, double-blind, controlled trial of sixty women in early pregnancy, more than 60% responded to a Seaband that pressed on an acupuncture point, while only 30% responded to the placebo band. [De Aloysio]

Patients often are nauseated after surgery, and one study of Seabands compared it to a placebo band and to an anti-emetic drug (one that prevents vomiting). The Seaband group had less nausea than either of the other groups. [Barsoum]

In a trial of more than a hundred people suffering from chemotherapy-induced nausea, more than three quarters of the subjects received some benefit from electrical stimulation (without needles) of P-6—an effect that could be prolonged by the use of Seabands. [Dundee] Another trial found that injecting a sugar solution into the P-6 point was as effective as an anti-emetic drug in preventing vomiting after surgery. [Yang]

Several studies didn't find a positive effect of P-6 stimulation. They include a double-blind trial of acupressure in the treatment of motion sickness, [Warwick-Evans] and a trial of children under anesthesia to determine whether P-6 acupuncture reduced postoperative vomiting. [Yentis] If the description of needle placement in the latter article is correct, the P-6 location was misidentified, which could certainly account for the negative result.

Substance abuse

Acupuncture is commonly used to help people withdraw from tobacco, alcohol, heroin or cocaine addiction; it's currently being studied by the National Institute of Drug Abuse, and it's used widely in New York City for outpatient drug detoxification. The points for treating drug addiction are found on the ear, and they can be taught relatively easily to laypeople, who then only use acupuncture for this specific purpose.

Detoxification from chronic use of prescribed opiates (morphine, Demerol, etc.) usually takes 3–6 months; even "brief" detoxification programs may take more than a month. In an uncontrolled trial of electrical stimulation at ear acupuncture points, twelve out of fourteen chronic pain patients (86%) were able to completely withdraw from narcotics within 2–7 days, and they experienced few or no side effects. [Kroening]

The evidence that acupuncture helps with withdrawal symptoms is tantalizing but insufficient, and it probably doesn't help prevent relapses at all. But given the dearth of successful medical treatments for addiction, there clearly needs to be more research into the role of acupuncture detoxification as part of a comprehensive treatment program.

An excellent review of studies of acupuncture and substance abuse was written by Brewington, Smith and Lipton, the first two of whom work at Lincoln Hospital in the Bronx, where the use of acupuncture in treating withdrawal symptoms of drug addiction was pioneered. If you're interested in a comprehensive analysis of both published and unpublished trials, see this review. [Brewington]

Regrettably, most of these studies weren't very well done. There were many methodological problems, and none of the eight trials on tobacco addiction they studied (which yielded mixed results) looked at whether acupuncture decreased withdrawal symptoms—which is what acupuncture is best for.

Lessening withdrawal symptoms is, unfortunately, only one aspect of ending an addiction, and acupuncture may not help in preventing a relapse. (When I was medical director of a clinic that did acupuncture detoxification, an acupuncturist there noticed that several of our clients clearly used acupuncture as a tune-up. Once they felt functional again, they went back to seeking drugs!)

There's surprisingly little research on cocaine addiction. However, one unpublished study described in the Brewington, Smith and Lipton review did find a better result for real acupuncture than sham acupuncture.

Two controlled studies on treatment of alcoholic recidivism—one with 80 patients and one with 54 patients—found that acupuncture treatment at fixed points was more effective than sham points in reducing expressed need for alcohol, drinking episodes, and hospital admissions for detoxification. But dropout rates were high, as they often are in substance abuse trials. [Bullock 1, Bullock 2]

A controlled study of real versus sham acupuncture in heroin detoxification found that addicts receiving the real treatment attended the acupuncture clinic more days and stayed in treatment longer. [Washburn] The treatment seemed to be most effective in those with lighter habits.

Several other studies found that acupuncture was equal to or better than methadone in helping people withdraw from heroin. [Man, Newmeyer] This is very important, because methadone treatment programs simply substitute a less expensive, longer-acting, government-sanctioned drug. Perhaps acupuncture, in combination with a relapse prevention program, could get addicts off both methadone and heroin.

Asthma and shortness of breath

Existing studies indicate that acupuncture is ineffective for long-term control of asthma, although a few studies show a modest temporary effect. One trial used a drug to induce an asthma attack, then compared real acupuncture to fake acupuncture, a placebo saline treatment and the drug isoproterenol. Real acupuncture worked better than fake acupuncture or the saline treatment, but isoproterenol worked best. [Tashkin 1]

Nineteen children with exercise-induced asthma were given either real or sham acupuncture. [Fung] Both groups improved, but those receiving real acupuncture improved more. Another controlled trial of 26 patients with disabling shortness of breath found that the real acupuncture group had less breathlessness and could walk further in six minutes than the sham acupuncture group. [Jobst]

Of thirteen controlled trials of acupuncture and asthma, eight had positive results while five were negative; a review found the positive effects of acupuncture on asthma unconvincing. [Kleijnen] Other trials found that acupuncture doesn't help exercise-induced asthma or moderate to severe asthma that's chronic. [Chow, Tashkin 2] One study in which seventeen patients were treated twice a week for five weeks found more improvement in the real acupuncture group after two weeks; after that, there was no difference between real and sham acupuncture. [Christensen 2]

Certainly the evidence is at best mixed, and any beneficial effect at best modest. Even if acupuncture does work temporarily for asthma, using it for an acute attack would be expensive and inconvenient.

Other uses of acupuncture

Acupuncture has been shown to improve neurological scores in stroke patients [Hu] and to increase maximum performance capacity and physical performance in young men. [Ehrlich] And electrical stimulation at acupuncture points has been found to increase uterine contractions in pregnant women who are past their due dates. [Dunn]

AYURVEDA AND YOGA

Ayurveda, which originated in India, is the oldest medical system known; its ancient texts cover all the major branches of medicine. [Sharma 3] Ayurveda is widely practiced in India and elsewhere. (There are other traditional Indian medical systems, less well-known in the United States, called Unani and Siddha.)

Ayurveda is Sanskrit for "the science (or knowledge) of life." It defines the trinity of life as body, mind and spiritual awareness, and is based on the concept of three *doshas*—physiological principles or bodily humors—called *vata, pitta* and *kapha.* (Together, they're called the *tridosha.)*

Each patient has a predominant dosha or combination of doshas; there are seven basic pure or mixed types. To an ayurvedic practitioner, imbalances in the doshas can cause specific diseases, and various foods and emotions can either stabilize or disturb the balance of a given dosha-type.

Ayurveda utilizes pulse and tongue diagnosis, diet, exercise and herbs. [Dash] A regimen called *panchakarma,* which means *five processes,* is often used for preventing disease. Oil massages and sweat baths precede an elimination regimen, which may include vomiting, purgatives, oil or herbal enemas, nasal cleansing and bloodletting. [Devaraj] Fasting, exercise, fresh air and hot herbs such as ginger and black pepper are often used after panchakarma. [Lad]

Some traditional ayurvedic medicines are made with dangerous heavy metals like lead and mercury.

It's claimed that heat-processing renders these medicines harmelss, but this hasn't been proven. Metal-
containing ayurvedic preparations should definitely
be avoided.

Two different types of ayurvedic medicine are practiced in the United States. Maharishi Ayur-Veda—started by Maharishi Mahesh Yogi, the Hindu swami best
known for popularizing Transcendental Meditation—
totally dominates traditional ayurveda. (For more
about TM, see the relaxation and meditation chapter.) Belonging to the same well-funded movement as
TM does, Maharishi Ayur-Veda markets an exclusive
line of products. [Skolnick] Most of the published studies
of ayurveda are on this version.

Herbs

Two Maharishi Ayur-Veda food supplements have
been studied in animals and cell cultures, but no ade-
quately designed studies on humans have been published. Both are herbal combinations claimed to be
based on traditional ayurvedic formulas, and are prepared with sweetened ghee (clarified butter).

Maharishi-4—also called Maharishi Amrit Kalash-4
or MAK-4—reduced the incidence of breast cancer in
rats. [Sharma 1] MAK-5 may also act to thin the blood—one
experiment showed that it prevented human platelet
aggregation in vitro. [Sharma 2] MAK-4 and MAK-5 may
also have antioxidant properties in vitro. [Niwa, Dwivedi]

Enemas in which sesame oil is retained are used in
ayurveda. One mediocre study shows that sesame oil
inhibits the growth of cultures of colon cancer cells,

37

but not more so than corn, soybean, safflower, olive and coconut oils. [Salerno]

The herb phyllanthus *(Phyllanthus amarus,* formerly *P. nituri)* is used in traditional ayurvedic, Chinese, African, South American, Central American and Caribbean medicine. A preliminary study treated 37 carriers of the hepatitis B virus with capsules of phyllanthus; 23 other carriers were given placebos. A month later, fewer than half of the treated group were still carrying the virus, while 96% of the control group were. [Thyagarajan]

A number of follow-up studies, however, have been unable to duplicate these results. [Unander] This is a good example of why it's important never to rely on a single study. Unless a study involves an extremely large number of subjects, it must be repeated before its results become credible.

In an uncontrolled study of 35 men, some with high and some with normal cholesterol, 50 grams of raw amla (the ayurvedic herb *Emblica officinalis,* also called *Indian gooseberry)* initially lowered cholesterol levels. But after a month, there was no significant reduction in either total or LDL cholesterol. [Jacob]

An uncontrolled study of 824 people with scabies was carried out in India. A paste of two herbs traditionally used for scabies and wounds—neem *(Azadirachta indica)* and turmeric *(Curcuma longa)*—was successful in 97% of the cases within three to fifteen days. [Charles]

Yoga

Yoga—the name means *union,* or *joining* in Sanskrit—is a sister-science to ayurveda; it's seen as important preventive medicine. Yoga is considered the science of the spirit and ayurveda the science of the body. Yogic postures *(asanas),* breathing exercises *(pranayama)* and forms of meditation have become popular in the United States. Yogic cleansing practices *(kriyas)* are practiced less often.

Most of the studies on yoga lack a control group or have other major flaws. The poor quality of these studies doesn't mean that yoga doesn't work, just that better studies should be done. In fact, there's a lot of anecdotal evidence that yoga has been very helpful to people.

A questionnaire distributed through national magazines asked people with chronic back pain to rate the treatments they'd tried; 492 self-selected readers responded. Moderate to dramatic long-term relief was reported by 23% of those who saw neurosurgeons, 28% of those who saw chiropractors, 65% of those who saw physical therapists and an amazing 96% of those who tried yoga! (the other 4% reported temporary relief). [Klein 1]

In a study of normal volunteers, yogic breathing exercises and stretching were compared with relaxation and visualization. [Wood] The yogic techniques produced greater increases in perceptions of mental and physical energy and enthusiasm than either of the other two interventions, but the results are too subjective to be very useful.

Some of the best studies examined a yogic technique that involves breathing through one nostril at a time. This has been shown (on an *electroencephalograph,* a machine that prints out recordings of brain waves called *EEGs)* to selectively stimulate the oppo-

39

site hemisphere of the brain. [Werntz] It's possible that it may also temporarily increase cognition in the opposite side of the brain, but studies on that effect have found mixed results. [Klein 2, Shanahoff-Khalsa]

A review of both published and unpublished studies found some evidence that yogic practices may be helpful in asthma. [Goyeche] In an uncontrolled study of 40 adolescent asthmatics, yoga training which included internal cleansing techniques (induced vomiting and diarrhea, and cleaning the nose and throat with salt water and a string) resulted in a significant increase in pulmonary function and exercise capacity; a two-year follow-up showed a good response, with reduced symptoms and reduced need for medication. [Jain 1]

An uncontrolled study of 149 diabetics concluded that yoga therapy decreased blood sugar and the use of diabetes medications. Unfortunately, this study was poorly designed—patients were placed on a vegetarian diet during it, and the changes in blood sugar may be simply due to that. [Jain 2]

An uncontrolled study of 20 patients with high blood pressure combined yogic relaxation, meditation and biofeedback work with a GSR meter (an instrument that measures *galvanic skin response*—the electrical resistance of the skin). The study found that 25% of the subjects were able to get off their hypertension medications, 35% were able to reduce them, 20% experienced better control of their blood pressure and only 20% didn't respond. [Patel]

BIOFEEDBACK

The will...is far less master of the mind than the body. A
man may resolve never to move from his chair, but he
cannot resolve never to be angry.

Peter Mere Latham (1789–1875) [Latham]

"I'll hold my breath till my face turns blue" is a threat
that parents can calmly ignore, because they know
that the breathing reflex will overcome even the most
stubborn child. But while we can't will our lungs to
stop, we *can* consciously affect many bodily processes
which might at first seem beyond our control. The
technology that lets you get on speaking terms with
parts of your body that you don't usually converse with
is called *biofeedback.*

Biofeedback equipment translates skin temperature, muscle contractions, blood pressure, pulse,
brain waves or other bodily functions into audio or
visual signals. By learning to control the pitch of a
sound, the rate of a series of beeps or an image on a
computer screen, you also learn to control the bodily
process that's being monitored. The patient is told to
use thoughts, feelings, sensations—whatever works to
affect the audio or visual signals in the appropriate
direction. Headaches, incontinence and even blood
flow are just a few of the physiological parameters that
can, with proper training, be influenced.

For example, people who have neck pain caused by
chronic muscle tension often benefit from *EMG (electromyographic)* biofeedback. Electrodes attached to
the neck muscles measure how tense they are, and the
monitoring equipment feeds that information back to
the subject by means of a beeping tone. (When the

muscles contract, the beeps get faster; when the muscles relax, the beeps get slower.) The people being trained do whatever's necessary to slow the beeping down. Once they've learned how to do that, they can then use the same technique to relax the muscles whenever they're tense.

Biofeedback differs from generalized relaxation in that you focus on a specific response—relaxing one muscle, say, or slowing your pulse—rather than trying to relax the whole body. General relaxation techniques may, of course, also slow the pulse, or relax the same specific muscle—in fact, they're almost certain to—but that's just a small part of the goal of relaxing the whole body. While distinct in their goals, biofeedback and relaxation techniques complement each other, and are often used together.

Many biofeedback practitioners don't consider biofeedback "alternative," because there's an enormous amount of scientific evidence backing its efficacy. It fits our definition, however, because it isn't routinely used in our current health care system.

Biofeedback helps a number of conditions for which conventional medicine has no good treatments, and it should be utilized in every clinic, hospital, and health practitioner's office. However, despite the documentation of its success for headache, incontinence, stroke rehabilitation and a host of other conditions, physicians rarely refer patients to biofeedback therapists. And insurance companies have been reluctant to pay for it.

While biofeedback training involves a therapist and specialized equipment, once the technique is learned, patients can use it anytime and anyplace. Perhaps it's this patient-controlled aspect that limits acceptance of biofeedback by the medical profession.

Headache

EMG biofeedback (often combined with relaxation) is very successful at treating headaches caused by muscle contraction. Its success rates—higher than those of medical or psychological treatments—range from 44% to 65%. [Andrasik] Biofeedback is even effective for patients whose muscle-contraction headaches are chronic and/or severe. [Bruhn]

There's also extensive data on the effectiveness of biofeedback for migraine headaches, which are caused by dilated blood vessels in the head. Biofeedback is used to teach patients how to warm their hands (by dilating the blood vessels in them). This affects blood flow to the head, thus reducing the pain. [Blanchard]

Circulation

Diabetics lose circulation in their feet, which can delay wound healing and increase the risk of amputation. Biofeedback-assisted relaxation may help avoid these complications. A study of 40 diabetics found that when patients used a general relaxation tape, they were able to increase their toe temperature 9%, but with biofeedback-assisted relaxation, they were able to increase it 31%. [Rice]

Stroke rehabilitation

EMG biofeedback is sometimes used to treat stroke patients with weakness on one side of their body. A meta-analysis that pooled data from eight controlled studies found that this approach helped improve patients' gait, grip, grasping ability and other hand functions. [Schleenbaker]

Urinary incontinence

Urinary incontinence is a widespread problem. One survey of almost 2000 people over 60 found that 19% of the men and 38% of the women suffered from it. [Diokno] The drugs used to treat this ailment have many side effects, and the conventional alternative—bladder suspension surgery—is a complicated operation that sometimes leaves the patient with difficulty urinating.

Most incontinence studies are uncontrolled. One study of 27 women found that after eight one-hour biofeedback sessions, 81% of the subjects were improved. [Cardozo] A trial of 64 women evaluated alternating biofeedback and intravaginal electrical stimulation. Almost two-thirds of the women improved—33% completely and 31% enough not to need further treatment. The remaining 36% didn't respond to the treatment. [Susset]

Another uncontrolled study of 48 incontinent women found that combining Kegel exercises (described in the exercise chapter) with biofeedback improved 62% of patients who came for two or more visits. [McIntosh] A larger, controlled study of 135 women compared Kegel exercises and biofeedback to an untreated control group. Urine losses were reduced 54% in the Kegel group and 61% in the biofeedback group; among the controls, it increased 9%. In the biofeedback group, 23% of the patients were completely cured vs. 16% in the Kegel group and 3% in the control group. [Burns]

Fecal incontinence

Fecal incontinence is also a widespread problem, affecting up to 1.5% of the general population [Whitehead] and 16% to 60% of the institutionalized elderly. [Brocklehurst] Besides its effect on one's social life, fecal incontinence can cause bladder infections and breakdown of the skin. Biofeedback training for this condition uses rectal balloons to train the patient to contract the anal sphincter in response to rectal distension.

In seven studies, this procedure resulted in complete elimination or markedly reduced frequency of fecal incontinence in 70% to 83% of patients. One to five treatments were required, and the beneficial effect was maintained at one- and two-year follow-ups. Although these studies were uncontrolled, many patients had been deemed incurable by conventional medical treatments, so the results are still impressive. [Marzuk]

A more recent study successfully treated liquid stool incontinence with biofeedback: twelve of sixteen patients with this problem improved significantly with biofeedback. [Chiarioni] Patients who are incontinent due to anorectal surgery seem to respond best to biofeedback training, but there is some evidence that diabetics with fecal incontinence also benefit. [Marzuk]

Alcoholism

Alcoholics hooked up to an *electroencephalograph* (a machine that produces brain-wave printouts called *EEGs)* can learn to increase the percentage of alpha

45

waves (associated with a relaxed state of mind) and theta waves (associated with deep meditation). A study found that depression scores dropped significantly with this treatment, compared to alcoholics who received daily therapeutic lectures and also to nonalcoholic controls. [Peniston 2]

Post-traumatic stress syndrome

A study found that Vietnam veterans with post-traumatic stress syndrome who received alpha-theta brainwave training were able to reduce their intake of psychiatric medications, compared to vets receiving conventional treatments. At a thirty-month follow-up, all fourteen control patients had relapsed, compared to only three of the fifteen vets who'd been taught the brainwave biofeedback. [Peniston 1]

Blood pressure

Biofeedback has only small effects on blood pressure. It can be effective for some patients with mild hypertension, but it doesn't work for everyone. [Glasgow] For people with moderate to severe hypertension, it isn't useful at all (fortunately, this condition can be successfully treated by drugs).

Other

Biofeedback has been shown to be more effective than acupuncture or drug treatment for chronic tinnitus (ringing in the ears), [Podoshin] more effective than relaxation and neck exercises for torticollis ("wry neck", which is caused by muscle spasms), [Jahanshahi] and more effective than exercises for chronic facial nerve paralysis. [Ross]

CHIROPRACTIC, ETC.

Therapeutic manipulation of the body has ancient roots: Hippocrates (fifth century BC), Aesklepiades (c. 100 BC) and Galen (second century AD) all used some form of it, and it was common among physicians until the eighteenth century. [Moore 1] The commonest forms of therapeutic manipulation practiced today—chiropractic and osteopathy—are the only major alternative therapies originally developed in the United States.

Chiropractic was invented by Daniel David Palmer, who was influenced by late-nineteenth-century spiritualism. Palmer performed his first spinal adjustment in September 1895, and claimed that he cured his patient—an African-American janitor—of deafness. The word *chiropractic,* coined by a patient a year later, comes from the Greek and means "done by hand."

Although Palmer was grandiose enough to date things *BC* ("before chiropractic") and *AC* ("after chiropractic"), osteopathy actually emerged before chiropractic. Andrew Taylor Still, the physician who originated osteopathy, began teaching his system in 1892, three years before Palmer's first adjustment.

Controversy still exists over whether chiropractic and osteopathy are twins separated at birth—or if chiropractic is the child of osteopathy. Palmer denied ever having met Dr. Still, but the two lived only about a day's journey from each other in the Midwest.

The two systems do differ somewhat in theory and practice. While osteopaths use arms and legs as fulcrums for bending and twisting the body *(long-lever manipulation),* chiropractors generally only manipulate the protruding parts of the spinal vertebrae *(short-lever manipulation).*

Similarities and differences aside, chiropractic has always dominated the field. Although osteopathy is a more complete system of medicine (doctors of osteopathy can perform surgery, prescribe drugs and do anything else medical doctors can do), chiropractors provide 94% of the manipulative therapy in the United States, and there's much more research on their work. [Shekelle 1]

Each year, 3–10% of the US population uses chiropractic services. A study conducted between 1974 and 1982 found that 7.5% of an insured population consulted a chiropractor in a given three-to-five-year period. [Shekelle 2] A 1980 report to Congress found that about 3.6% of the population visited chiropractors each year. [Von Kuster] A Harvard telephone survey found that 10% of the population used chiropractic in 1990. [Eisenberg]

Women have been trained in chiropractic from its inception. Three of the first "Fifteen Disciples" of D.D. Palmer's Chiropractic School and Cure were women— one of whom, Minora Paxson, coauthored the first chiropractic textbook. By the 1920s, between a third and a half of chiropractors were women.

(As late as the 1930s, only about 5% of medical school graduates were female. But even fewer went on to practice as doctors, because they were denied the internships they needed. On average, 185 internships were available to the 250 women who graduated medical school each year, while more than 6000 internships were open to the fewer than 5000 male graduates.) [Walsh]

The percentage of women chiropractors dropped precipitously after World War II. In one representative school, 22 out of 36 students who graduated between 1943 and 1945 were women, while of the 90 who graduated in 1949, only three were. In the fifties and sixties, no more than four women graduated in any class. [Moore 3]

Only in the last thirty years has the number of female chiropractors increased, and even that increase has been modest; in 1994, women still accounted for only 12% of the profession. [ACA]

While the end of WWII was disastrous for women in chiropractic, it seemed at first to be a boon for African-Americans. Many chiropractic schools, spurred by the prospect of cashing in on the educational benefits of the GI Bill, opted for desegregation; in addition, several black chiropractic colleges were founded.

But of the three schools catering specifically to African-American veterans, two closed shortly after the 1951 deadline for veterans' educational benefits. [Moore 2] Enrollment also dropped dramatically in the other chiropractic schools, and has never recovered; in 1994, only 1% of chiropractors were African-Americans. [ABCA]

Unsurprisingly, awareness of the benefits of chiropractic is also low in the African-American community. A survey conducted in St. Louis in the early 1980s found that 78% of African-American residents had experienced back pain, but only 1% had ever visited a chiropractor. [Moore 2]

49

MDs vs. chiropractors

The medical profession has been consistently and relentlessly hostile to chiropractic. In Abraham Flexner's famous 1910 report on the state of medical education, chiropractic is dismissed without consideration. Standards were low for admission to both chiropractic and medical schools at the time. Standards for both rose by 1930, and many inferior medical and chiropractic schools folded at that time. [Moore 4]

In 1962, the general counsel of the Iowa Medical Society, Robert B. Throckmorton, formulated a plan to "contain" chiropractic in the state by encouraging "ethical" complaints against chiropractors and opposing the coverage of chiropractic services by health insurance, worker's compensation or labor unions. In 1963, the American Medical Association invited Throckmorton to implement chiropractic containment nationwide, and its board of trustees voted to establish a Committee on Chiropractic—whose name was soon changed to the Committee on Quackery—that considered its "prime mission to be, first, the containment" and "ultimately the elimination of chiropractic."

In 1966, the AMA House of Delegates adopted a resolution to ensure that physicians understood that they were forbidden to associate with chiropractors. The Judicial Council ruled that a doctor would be guilty of unethical conduct if he or she even lectured to a group of chiropractors on a medical subject. One member of the Committee on Quackery told a workshop of the Michigan State Medical Society that a medical doctor would be acting unethically if he or she referred a patient to a chiropractor for any reason.

In answer to questions from physicians as to whether they had to resign from Rotary Clubs and other civic organizations that chiropractors also belonged to, the Judicial Council stated that resignation would be necessary if the organization involved itself directly or indirectly with health care concerns. [ACA] In the early 1970s, the Joint Commission on the Accreditation of Hospitals informed hospital administrators that if chiropractors were granted privileges, accreditation would be withdrawn, even if state legislation required hospitals to accept chiropractors as members of the hospital staff!

In 1976, Chester Wilk and four fellow chiropractors filed an antitrust suit against the AMA, the American Hospital Association, the American Academy of Orthopaedic Surgeons, five other medical associations and four individuals, alleging a conspiracy to eliminate chiropractic through refusal to associate professionally with chiropractors. In 1987, the AMA and its codefendants were found guilty of boycott and conspiracy, and a permanent injunction was issued preventing the AMA from restricting association with chiropractors. The AMA appealed the decision, but lost in 1990. [Moore 8]

Despite the enmity of the medical community, consumers have been very supportive of chiropractic, and in 1974, Congress passed legislation requiring Medicare to pay for chiropractic services. In the same year, two million dollars were allocated to the National Institutes of Health for scientific study of the biomechanics of chiropractic manipulation; authorization was granted for accreditation of chiropractic colleges; and the last two holdout states granted licenses to chiropractors. [Moore 7] Today, about 85% of insurance companies cover chiropractic services. [ACA]

Osteopathic physicians learn both conventional medicine and manipulation techniques. (They're usually called *DO's,* which is short for *doctors of osteopathy.)* Trained in a more "holistic" fashion than MD's, some DO's stay true to their roots, while others go out of their way to be as MD-like as possible—even to the extent of not incorporating osteopathic manipulation into their practices.

There are more osteopaths than MD's in primary-care medicine (which is more generalist, front-line and cost-effective than medical specialities). Almost half of all DO's are in general or family practice, and another 20% or so are in pediatrics or internal medicine. They also tend to be younger than MD's—half of all DO's graduated in the last ten years. However, while the number of women DO's doubled between 1989 and 1995, they still make up only a quarter of the field—about the same measly proportion as among MD's. [AOA]

Back pain
Evidence for the clinical effectiveness of spinal adjustment has been gathering since about 1952. A Harvard survey found that the most common reason for seeking chiropractic treatment is back pain, and that a fifth of back pain sufferers have used chiropractic. [Eisenberg]

A 1974 retrospective study of back pain patients who'd received workman's compensation found that patients were equally happy—and equally improved—with chiropractic as with medical treatment. [Kane] Twelve years later, a study of back pain patients enrolled in a health maintenance organization made the same comparison and found that three times as many patients were satisfied with chiropractic care as with medical treatment. [Cherkin] Either patients are becoming more enthusiastic about chiropractic or more disenchanted with their physicians.

Although there are numerous studies of spinal adjustment, most are small and not well controlled. However, there are fortunately some exceptions. In what is widely considered to be one of the best studies, Hadler compared the effects of a single long-lever manipulation with those of mobilization (described below) on 54 patients with acute low-back pain. He found that among patients who'd had backache for more than two weeks, those who received the real manipulation improved faster than the controls. [Hadler]

In a 1955 study, credited as the first controlled trial of spinal manipulation, a technique called *Cyriax manipulation* (sort of a nonspecific osteopathic manipulation) was compared to a combination of bed rest, a lumbar pillow and painkillers. At the end of a week, 50% of the manipulated patients were free of signs and symptoms, compared with 27% of the control group. At the end of six weeks, only 12% of the manipulated group had signs and symptoms, while 28% of the control group was still suffering. [Coyer]

An assessment in Oregon of 237 workman's compensation claims for back pain found that 82% of the

29 workers treated only by a chiropractor resumed work after one week without a disability award. Only 41% of claimants treated solely by a medical doctor went back to work after one week. [Moore 5]

A study of one thousand back injury reports recorded at the California Division of Labor Statistics and Research found that the five hundred patients who received chiropractic care lost less time and were more likely to report complete recovery than those who had only medical care. [Moore 6]

Another trial, involving 95 patients, taught all of them back care and exercises; half the group also received manipulation. There was some advantage for manipulated patients one to two weeks after the commencement of treatment, but at four weeks the two groups were equivalent. [MacDonald]

Another study found no benefit of chiropractic over "back school"—that is, instruction in back exercises and avoiding back stress (posture and proper lifting). [Bergquist-Ullmann] One study compared painkillers, corset use, physical therapy and chiropractic and found no advantage to manipulation. [Doran]

Another trial of 256 patients with nonspecific back and neck complaints divided patients into four groups—those receiving chiropractic adjustments, physical therapy (exercise, massage, heat, ultrasound or low-level electricity treatments), continued treatment by the general practitioner or a placebo treatment. Chiropractic produced a faster and larger improvement in physical functioning than the other three therapies, but changes in spinal mobility weren't consistent. [Koes 2]

A meta-analysis of nine high-quality studies of spinal manipulation for low-back pain found a definite improvement at three weeks for patients who had uncomplicated, acute pain. For patients with chronic pain, or pain with sciatic nerve irritation, the data were less clear. [Shekelle 2] Two other meta-analyses found only limited support for spinal manipulation and mobilization. [Ottenbacher, Koes 1]

Not surprisingly, a meta-analysis published in the chiropractic literature is more supportive. Drawing on 23 randomized controlled trials of spinal manipulation for back pain, this analysis found that spinal manipulation was more effective than any comparison treatment. [Anderson] The federal government agrees—at least as far as acute back pain goes. In 1994, the federal Agency for Health Care Policy and Research released a guideline endorsing the use of chiropractic for acute low-back pain. The agency found that the evidence concerning chronic back pain was mixed, and only endorsed chiropractic for acute back pain. [Bigos]

Mobilization

Although definitions vary, manipulation and mobilization (which is used mostly by physical therapists) are generally distinguished from one another by the extent of movement. Mobilization moves a joint just until resistance is felt, whereas manipulation takes the joint to its full anatomic limit, beyond which injury would occur. [Raftis]

Maitland mobilization is a gentle, long-lever approach that involves rotatory movements along the spine. It's been found to hasten improvement in outpatients with nonspecific back pain, but not to affect their long-term prognosis. [Sims-Williams 2] In a randomized study of 741 patients with low-back pain, those treated by chiropractors scored 7% better on pain and functioning scales at a two-year follow-up than those given Maitland mobilization by the hospital staff. Patients treated by chiropractors also lost fewer days of work. [Meade]

For sciatica, Maitland mobilization was slightly better than traction, exercise or corseting in the short term, but there was no long-term benefit for any of the treatments. [Coxhead]

Eighty-four patients with back pain were randomly given either a single rotatory mobilization by a physical therapist or a treatment with a deactivated heat therapy machine. Patients treated with the mobilization reported more relief from pain than the control group fifteen minutes after the treatment, but there was no difference between the two groups at three and seven days. (This may simply mean that adequate treatment would have required more than one manipulation.) [Glover]

Other back pain therapies

In patients referred to specialist clinics for back pain, Maitland mobilization showed no definite advantage over placebo physical therapy. This may not have been the best study, because the placebo used was low-level microwave radiation, which is hardly a placebo at all, since it might very well have some effect on pain. [Sims-Williams 1]

A single-blind trial of 81 adults suffering from recent low-back pain compared superficial massage, low-level electrostimulation and a rotational technique called *Maigne manipulation* (high-velocity, localized thrusts, similar to osteopathic manipulations but in the opposite direction). All three groups showed improvement. (Again, low-level electrostimulation may help with pain, so it doesn't seem the best choice for a placebo control.) [Godfrey]

A trial comparing heat treatment with manipulation found the latter helpful only in a subgroup of patients who had limited ability to pass a basic diagnostic test for back pain. [Mathews]

Slipped disks
For patients with slipped disks, chiropractic does nothing to affect the extent of disk protrusion but it does help to alleviate pain. [Wilson, Chrisman] That's not surprising, since the extent to which a disk bulges or protrudes may have nothing to do with the severity of pain. In one of my favorite studies, *MRI* (magnetic resonance imaging) was used to examine 98 people without back pain; 52% of the subjects had a bulge at one or more vertebral levels, and only 36% of these pain-free people had normal disks at all levels! [Jensen]

Other conditions
Does spinal adjustment help problems other than back pain? There are only a few satisfactory studies on the effectiveness of chiropractic for other conditions. One study of migraine patients found that both chiropractic

manipulation and cervical mobilization reduced the frequency and duration of migraines, but that chiropractic manipulation was superior for pain reduction. [Parker] A controlled study of 29 patients with high blood pressure found no effect on the condition. [Morgan]

A comparison of chiropractic manipulation with a sham manipulation for menstrual cramps showed that the real thing was twice as likely to alleviate cramps and discomfort. [Kokjohn] A small dysmenorrhea (menstrual cramps) trial provided chiropractic manipulation to eight women, while three controls went untreated. Seven of the eight women treated with manipulation at least twice a week experienced decreased pain and disability, while none of the controls did. [Thomason]

An uncontrolled trial of 316 infants with colic found that chiropractic manipulation produced improvement in 94% of cases. Two weeks after the beginning of treatment, the average length of a colic episode had decreased by 75%. Many of the babies had been previously treated, unsuccessfully, with medication or diet change. [Klougart] A valuable follow-up to this study would be a controlled trial in which chiropractic manipulation was compared with simethicone, the most common treatment for colic.

A study of 46 bed-wetting children compared chiropractic adjustment with a sham adjustment and found that although the children who received the real adjustments improved, the results weren't statistically significant. [Reed]

For asthma, a crossover trial compared real and sham chiropractic treatment on 31 patients (each patient receiving twice-weekly real or sham treatments for four weeks, then crossing over to the other group). No significant difference was found between the two treatments. [Nielsen]

Adverse effects

The total number of complications due to spinal manipulation reported in the English, French and German literature from 1900 to 1980 is 135—a minuscule number given the widespread use of chiropractic. Complications from manipulation of the cervical (neck) vertebrae are also extremely rare—just 54 cases of stroke and other neurovascular incidents. [Laderman]

Manipulation of the lumbar region (lower back) seems to be even safer. There are only about 29 cases reported of the most-feared complication, cauda equina syndrome, and 16 of those occurred during manipulation under anesthesia, a technique no longer used. *(Cauda equina* means *horse's tail* and refers to the bundle of nerves that hangs from the spinal cord below the protection of the vertebra. Damage to these nerves can cause numbness or paralysis in the lower limbs.) The frequency of cauda equina syndrome is estimated to be on the order of one per hundred million lower-back manipulations. [Shekelle 1]

Conclusion

Chiropractic *is* demonstrably beneficial for acute low-back pain, but its effect on chronic back pain is less dramatic (although other forms of manipulation also have some benefit for back pain). While the jury's still out on the long-term benefits of chiropractic treatment, shortening an episode of acute back pain is no small matter. The difference between being flat on your back for two weeks or six is a month of your life.

Back pain is a major public health problem, and benign methods of treatment are sorely needed. However, more research is required to establish exactly which groups of people with back pain benefit most.

In spite of the inconclusiveness of the data, consumers are voting with their feet—or, more accurately, with their backs—in their enthusiastic use of chiropractors. I regularly refer patients to chiropractors for backache, neck pain, and occasionally for recalcitrant headaches—with positive results. There's little evidence, however, that spinal manipulation can cure internal disease, and any such claims should be met with skepticism.

DIETARY SUPPLEMENTS AND NUTRITON

Dietary changes and nutritional supplements won't make it possible for us to live forever, but they'll probably help prolong our lives, and they're even more likely to help us stay healthy until as late in life as possible. Not only can small amounts of a vitamin or mineral greatly benefit a person suffering from a deficiency disease, but in many cases they'll also help someone whose diet isn't clearly deficient.

Controversy persists about whether supplements can prevent and treat diseases, and they're still underused for those purposes. Aging appears to increase the need for certain vitamins, and the FDA's recommended daily allowances *(RDAs)* may be too low for vitamin D, riboflavin, vitamin B_6 and B_{12} in elderly people. For vitamin A, however, the RDA may be too high. [Russell]

Discussions of about twenty types of nutrients and supplements follow below, in alphabetical order.

Antioxidants
Antioxidants are nutrients that protect against *oxidation,* a chemical reaction which can do profound damage to the cells of our bodies. Antioxidants include vitamins A, C and E, beta-carotene and other carotenoids, flavonoids and the mineral selenium.

Many physicians believe in the power of antioxidants. At a meeting of 700 cardiologists, roughly two-thirds raised their hands when asked whether they took antioxidants. [Jancin]

61

All the antioxidant nutrients are discussed in their own sections below. In addition, some of the results described in the multivitamins section are no doubt due to the effects of the antioxidants.

Amino acids

Amino acids, the building blocks of proteins, can have pronounced drug-like effects when taken singly, and should be taken with as much caution as drugs. Some of these effects are beneficial, but amino acids aren't entirely benign substances.

In a placebo-controlled study of 31 men with untreated coronary artery disease, a stress test was given. (In a *stress test,* the patient exercises while hooked up to an EKG. *EKG* stands for *electrocardiogram*—that is, a heart monitor. Why the *K?* Because the original name for the device was German.)

The stress test was then repeated after intravenous injection of either the amino acid carnitine (in the form of L-propionylcarnitine) or a placebo. The group that got the carnitine had fewer changes in their EKG, and their hearts pumped more efficiently. [Bartels]

A double-blind trial of 44 men with chronic, stable *angina* (chest pains caused by the heart not getting enough oxygen) found similar results: when they took L-carnitine pills, 48% of the men increased their maximum exercise work load, compared to 11% during the placebo phase. Also, fewer EKG changes were noted during the carnitine portion of the experiment. [Cherchi]

Another trial of heart attack patients compared 79 subjects who took conventional medication with 81 subjects who also took carnitine. The carnitine group's heart rates improved, and they had fewer anginal attacks and a lower death rate (1.2% vs. 12.5% in the control group). [Davini]

A double-blind, crossover study of 20 patients with intermittent claudication (a circulatory problem that causes pain in the legs during exercise)) found that those treated with carnitine could walk almost twice as far as those treated with a placebo. [Brevetti] L-carnitine seems safe; DL-carnitine can cause muscle weakness in some people.

Another amino acid, tryptophan, had been used for depression and insomnia, but it's no longer sold in the US because a batch contaminated with an unknown substance caused about 1500 cases of a debilitating condition called eosinophilia-myalgia syndrome, and about 40 deaths. There's some evidence that, in combination with other treatments, tryptophan may help depression, but a review of tryptophan trials found that it's unsuccessful as a treatment by itself. [Chouinard]

Lysine is often used to treat or prevent herpes infections, but there are fewer positive trials [Kagan, Griffith] than negative ones, [Milman 1 & 2, DiGiovanna] and the negative ones are better. There's actually a sound physiological basis for lysine to work, but when it's studied in a controlled manner, it doesn't seem to.

Beta-carotene and other carotenoids

An excess of vitamin A—or of its derivatives, like retinoic acid—can cause headaches, nausea, itchy skin, brittle nails, liver toxicity, bone pain and birth defects. Beta-carotene *metabolizes* (changes) into vitamin A in our bodies, but it's impossible to take a toxic dose of it, because your body simply won't convert enough of it into vitamin A. All too much beta-carotene will do is turn your palms—and, later, the rest of your skin—orange.

In addition to being less toxic, beta-carotene is also a stronger antioxidant than vitamin A. In a case-controlled study of 191 pairs of women in Italy, those whose diets provided the least beta-carotene had six times the risk of developing invasive cervical cancer than those who consumed the most. [LaVecchia]

One study found that high levels of beta-carotene in the blood protected strongly against a type of lung cancer called squamous-cell carcinoma. [Menkes] In another study, 683 people who'd had heart attacks had lower levels of beta-carotene in their fat tissue than 727 controls. [Kardinaal]

While these studies show that people who eat foods high in beta-carotene have lower risk of various diseases, results have been disappointing when the beta-carotene comes in pill form. Beta-carotene is one of a class of related compounds called *carotenoids,* and the benefits of the foods that are high in beta-carotene may actually be due more to the other *carotenoids*—or to other, as-yet-unidentified substances that also tend to be present when beta-carotene is.

This may be why a notorious study of Finnish smokers found that those who took beta-carotene supplements had a death rate from lung cancer that was 8% *higher* than the control group. [ABCPSG] Although it wasn't published by the time this book went to press, another large trial—called, cutely enough, the CARET study—has confirmed the negative effect of beta carotene in smokers.

B vitamins

Vitamins B_1 *(thiamine)*, B_2 *(riboflavin)*, B_3 *(niacin)* and B_6 *(pyridoxine)* are *co-enzymes,* which means they're needed by enzymes to carry out many biochemical functions. *(Enzymes* are proteins that catalyze biochemical reactions.) B_1 is necessary for energy production and the transmission of signals down the nerves; it also helps protect against alcohol-induced damage. B_2, B_3 and B_6 regulate the synthesis of a number of hormones.

Vitamin B_{12} *(cobalamin)* and folic acid (or *folate,* which is also a B vitamin) maintain the health of nerve cells and are necessary for the formation of red blood cells and DNA. The body also requires vitamins B_{12}, B_6 and folate to rid itself of a substance called *homocysteine.* A derivative of methionine, an amino acid found mainly in animal products, homocysteine can accumulate in the blood, and has been linked to an increased risk of cardiovascular disease, [Stampfer 2, Israelsson] stroke, [Coull] miscarriages and certain birth defects.

Twenty-one percent of women with recurrent unexplained miscarriages had elevated homocysteine levels. [Wouters] as did mothers of babies born with neural tube birth defects like spina bifida ("split spine") and anencephaly (in which the baby is born missing most of its brain). [Mills]

Folic acid, which is known to lower homocysteine levels, [Selhub] dramatically lowers the rate of neural tube defects, but it must be taken very early in pregnancy to be effective. Vitamin B_{12} may also help to lower the risk of neural tube defects. [Mills]

Unfortunately, few Americans eat enough fresh fruits and vegetables, the dietary sources of folic acid. One study found that 13%–15% of women 20–44 years of age showed biochemical evidence of folate deficiency. [Senti]

Supplements can help make up for this. In one study, adding folate, B_6 and B_{12} to the diets of 22 men reduced their homocysteine levels by more than half. Some of the men were then able to keep their homocysteine down by diet alone; in others, it rose to its previous level. [Ubbink]

Every man, woman and fetus should have a daily dose of folic acid. Besides decreasing homocysteine levels and spina bifida rates, it may also decrease the rate of cardiovascular disease, colon cancer and cervical cancer.

Unfortunately, the Food and Drug Administration currently restricts the dosage of folic acid pills to 800 micrograms (a *microgram* is a thousandth of a milligram). Dosages of a milligram or higher are available only by prescription, even in prenatal vitamin formulas.

The FDA's rationale for this restriction is that a dose of over one milligram could prevent a certain blood test from detecting pernicious anemia, which is caused by a deficiency of either folic acid or B_{12}. If a person suffering from pernicious anemia caused by a B_{12} deficiency took a large dose of folic acid, the anemia blood test wouldn't detect the B_{12} deficiency.

However, measuring serum B_{12} levels is a more specific, more effective way to determine B_{12} deficiency. The commonly available serum B_{12} test isn't done often enough.

There's some evidence that folic acid may compromise the effectiveness of certain drugs, including methotrexate, colchicine, trimethoprim and phenytoin. [Butterworth 1] Extremely large doses may interfere with zinc metabolism, but the studies on this show conflicting results. There are several case reports of hypersensitivity to folic acid in doses of one to ten milligrams, but such reports are very rare, and may be due to other ingredients in the supplements.

A high intake of dietary folate (the natural form of folic acid) protects against *colorectal adenoma,* a precancerous condition that can lead to colon cancer. [Giovannucci] Low folate intake also increases risk for another precancerous condition called cervical dysplasia. (Although cervical cancer appears to be caused by a sexually transmitted virus, a deficiency of folate appears also to be a factor.) [Butterworth 2] Folinic acid, a type of folate, has been used successfully to treat a type of male infertility called round cell idiopathic syndrome. [Bentivoglio]

Folic acid and vitamin B_{12} often work together. One small but interesting, uncontrolled Argentinian study of *vitiligo* (a skin disease characterized by whitish nonpigmented areas surrounded by hyperpigmented borders) found that supplementation of eight subjects with folic acid, vitamin B_{12} and vitamin C resulted in noticeable repigmentation. [Montes]

B_{12} may have other uses as well. In one study of military personnel, almost half of subjects with tinnitus (ringing in the ears) and noise-induced hearing loss were found to be deficient in vitamin B_{12}. [Shemesh] And a case series of five asthmatic children who were sensitive to sulfites found that vitamin B_{12} prevented an asthmatic attack in four of them. [Anibarro]

Because niacin (vitamin B_3) reduces triglycerides and *LDL* (low-density lipoprotein, the "bad" cholesterol) and increases *HDL* (high-density lipoprotein, the "good" cholesterol), it's sometimes used in conventional medicine for these purposes. [Christensen, Alderman]

In a trial of 124 subjects with intermittent claudication (described above in the *amino acids* section), 72% of those receiving inositol nicotinate, a derivative of niacin, reported improvement, compared to 45% of subjects who got a placebo. [O'Hara]

Unfortunately, niacin is the B vitamin with the most side effects, both minor and severe. Besides causing flushing, nausea, diarrhea, headache and fatigue, it can also be toxic to the liver—especially in its sustained-release form. One study found signs of liver toxicity in half the subjects taking sustained-release niacin, but none in those taking immediate-release niacin. [McKenney]

In a study of 59 pregnant women, vitamin B_6 (pyridoxine) was more effective than a placebo in reducing severe nausea and vomiting caused by pregnancy (no difference was found in mild to moderate nausea). [Sahakian] This is interesting, because the only medication ever approved by the FDA for that problem was Bendectin, a mixture of vitamin B_6 and a drug called doxylamine.

Bendectin was later removed from the market by the manufacturer because of lawsuits alleging that it caused birth defects. (This was never proven, but multiple lawsuits made the drug unprofitable.)

B_6—which has been used for morning sickness since at least 1942—may have been the active ingredient in Bendectin, and it's never been implicated in birth defects on its own. [Willis] However, taking more than 100 mgs of B_6 a day can cause insomnia or other problems.

Calcium

Calcium is a mineral needed for normal muscle and nerve function, as well as for the development and maintenance of bones and teeth. There's conflicting evidence as to whether or not dietary calcium lowers blood pressure. Among 25 observational studies, most found that it did, but out of nineteen randomized controlled trials testing the effect of calcium supplementation on blood pressure, eleven showed no significant effect, only two showed a significant effect, and the rest were equivocal. [Cutler]

One review found that calcium reduced the blood pressure of hypertensives in twelve studies, but seven other studies found no decrease. [Mikami] A review of 24 published studies found that overall, calcium reduced blood pressure in at least part of the study population, but thirteen of the studies found no difference. [Hatton]

It's possible that calcium may be most important in reducing blood pressure in certain subsets of the hypertensive population—African-Americans, salt-sensitive individuals and women with preeclampsia (hypertension induced by pregnancy, which can be life-threatening both for women and their fetuses). One study of 1194 pregnant women found that those given calcium had a 37% reduction in preeclampsia. [Belizan]

While existing data doesn't support the use of calcium as a routine hypertension treatment, some individuals with mild hypertension may have good results with it. More research should be done on the effect of calcium on various subsets of the hypertensive population.

A small study of ten subjects found that calcium helps normalize the *mucosa* (mucous membrane) of the colon in people at high risk of developing colon cancer. [Lipkin]

Calcium can cause constipation and, in large amounts, a condition called milk-alkali syndrome that raises calcium levels in the blood to dangerously high levels. The citrate portion of calcium citrate (an easily absorbable, popular form of calcium) may increase absorption of aluminum from food and water—probably not something you want to do. [Nolan]

Many calcium supplements—particularly those made from bonemeal, dolomite or "natural sources" (usually limestone derived from fossilized oyster shells)—contain a significant amount of lead. [Bourgoin] (Refined or chelated calcium has the least lead.) Even milk isn't lead-free, although the levels it contains are low and are generally deemed "acceptable."

Coenzyme Q$_{10}$

Coenzyme Q$_{10}$ is an essential part of mitochondria, the energy-producing part of cells. (Typically abbreviated CoQ_{10}, it's also called *ubiquinone,* because it's found in virtually every cell of the body.) Diseased hearts tend to have less CoQ_{10} in them, and supplementation with CoQ_{10} appears to be beneficial in various types of heart disease.

In a randomized, double-blind, controlled trial of 641 patients with congestive heart failure, patients receiving CoQ_{10} required fewer hospitalizations and had fewer serious complications. [Morisco] And a small, controlled study showed that exercise tolerance increased in twelve angina patients treated with CoQ_{10}. [Kamikawa]

In people who've undergone coronary artery bypass operations, CoQ_{10} protects hearts from postoperative complications. In a controlled trial, 40 patients received CoQ_{10} or a placebo for a week prior to their operation. The blood tests of treated subjects showed less evidence of heart injury than commonly occurs after this operation, and the treated group also had a lower incidence of arrhythmias during the recovery period. [Chello]

Copper

Our bodies need copper, a heavy metal, to make the oxygen-carrying hemoglobin in our red blood cells. However, copper is toxic in large amounts—over 35 mg a day or so. (Two mgs a day or less should be safe, but most people don't need supplemental copper at all.) In a study of 1666 Finnish men, those with the highest amounts of copper in their blood had a risk of heart attack four times higher than those with the lowest amounts. [Salonen]

71

Chromium

The body needs chromium to regulate blood sugar, and it may also increase HDL (described above). That was the finding of a study of 72 men who were receiving beta blockers for hypertension and took 600 micrograms of chromium daily for two months. [Roeback] Chromium may also increase glucose tolerance, although it's not clear that it helps people who are already diabetic.

Fish and fish oil

There's evidence that eating fish or taking fish oil supplements can benefit a wide variety of problems, including high blood pressure, clogged arteries, pulmonary disease, rheumatoid arthritis, kidney disease, eczema, psoriasis, premature birth, cystic fibrosis and ulcerative colitis. There aren't any known adverse effects (except possibly bad breath), and overdoses are very unlikely. In fact, fairly large quantities of capsules must be taken (most studies used ten to eighteen grams a day), or oily fish—such as salmon, mackerel, sardines or bluefish—must be eaten at least three times weekly.

The arteries of patients who've undergone coronary angioplasty ("roto-rooting" of the blood vessels supplying the heart) often close up again. A meta-analysis of seven trials on these patients found that fish oil reduced the rate at which the treated arteries clogged up again. In four studies in which pictures of the arteries were taken, the difference between the placebo and fish oil groups was 14%. The more fish oil people ingested, the greater the effect. [Gapinski]

Eating fish thins the blood, which may also be how fish oil helps arteries. A large, population-based study found that people who ate fish once or more a day had the fewest clotting factors in their blood. [Shahar 2] Fish in the diet also is associated with less risk of chronic obstructive pulmonary disease (emphysema or chronic bronchitis) in smokers. [Shahar 1]

In a meta-analysis of 31 trials on 1356 subjects, fish oil reduced blood pressure in hypertensive people, but not in those whose blood pressure was normal. [Morris]

Fish oil helps rheumatoid arthritis symptoms, perhaps because of its apparent anti-inflammatory effects. In one study, 64 subjects received fish oil or a placebo; after three months, the fish oil group was able to reduce their intake of painkilling drugs significantly. [Lau] Another controlled trial of 51 subjects with active rheumatoid arthritis found that those who took fish oil had a significant reduction in morning stiffness and joint stiffness; however, there were no significant changes in joint swelling, pain level, grip strength or daily activity level. [Nielson]

Another trial of 37 subjects gave one group fish oil along with a diet high in polyunsaturated fat and low in saturated fat; the control group took a placebo along with a diet with a higher ratio of saturated to polyunsaturated fat. The results were similar to the previous trial; at a three-month follow-up examination, the fish oil group had less morning stiffness and fewer tender joints. [Kremer]

Another double-blind trial of 60 patients with rheumatoid arthritis compared fish oil to olive oil.

Morning stiffness and pain improved in both groups, but an improvement in tender joints and grip strength occurred only in the fish oil group. [Cleland]

A trial of 49 subjects tested evening primrose oil (EPO) against a combination of fish oil and EPO (both sources of essential fatty acids) and against a placebo. Both treated groups had significant subjective improvement and lowered their usage of painkillers. [Belch] (For more on EPO, see the herbs chapter.)

Fish oil also slows a common type of kidney disease called IgA nephropathy. In one trial, 55 subjects taking fish oil capsules lost kidney function more slowly than 51 subjects taking a placebo. [Donadio] This is particularly exciting since various drug therapies have failed to help this disease.

Sixty-six kidney transplant patients were divided into two groups: one got six grams of fish oil daily, the other got coconut oil. After a year, the fish oil patients had better functioning kidneys and fewer rejection episodes (although there was no difference in the survival rate of kidneys between the groups). [van der Heide]

The evidence on whether fish oil helps psoriasis is mixed. Several studies note improvement, [Bittiner, Maurice, Lassus] but at least one double-blind study found no difference from a placebo. [Soyland]

Similarly, there are conflicting results from several studies on the effect of fish oil in treating eczema. [Bjorneboe, Kunz] A recent, placebo-controlled trial of fish oil and EPO found that neither helped eczema. [Berth-Jones]

Fish oil may become an important tool in preventing premature birth, and it can also benefit premature babies. A study of 533 pregnant Danish women found that those who were given fish oil capsules had longer pregnancies than those who got olive oil capsules. [Olsen] In other research, the vision of healthy premature babies who were given fish oil improved more than that of babies in a control group. [Carlson]

In a trial of eighteen patients with ulcerative colitis, patients took fish oil or a placebo for four months, then crossed over to the other treatment. Fish oil improved the appearance of tissue under a microscope, and enabled patients to gain weight (both positive signs for sufferers of this ailment). [Stenson]

Finally, in cystic fibrosis patients, fish oil improved lung function. (Cystic fibrosis is a serious genetic disease in which mucus clogs the lungs.) [Lawrence]

Flavonoids

Vitamins and minerals aren't the only kinds of antioxidants. Flavonoids are a large class of antioxidants found in fruits, vegetables, tea and wine. In vitro, they appear to inhibit the oxidation of LDL ("bad" cholesterol) and to reduce the formation of blood clots. One study of the diets of men over 65 found that the higher the intake of flavonoids, the lower the mortality from coronary heart disease. [Hertog 2]

While there haven't been prospective trials on humans, there does seem to be a correlation between dietary intake of flavonoids and lowered cardiovascular disease in humans. In 805 men over 65 followed from 1985 to 1990, the more flavonoids consumed, the fewer number of heart attacks. [Hertog 2] In fact, those who consumed the most flavonoids had a heart attack rate less than half that of those who consumed the fewest. The most common dietary sources of flavonoids for subjects in the study were tea (61%), onions (13%) and apples (10%).

Another study by the same investigator looked at whether flavonoid intake could explain differences in mortality rates in seven countries. He found that flavonoid consumption could explain about a quarter of the difference in heart disease rate, but that it didn't seem to have any correlation with cancer rates. [Hertog 1]

Iodine

Iodine is necessary for normal thyroid function. *Goiters* (swollen thyroid glands that protrude from the neck) and *cretinism* (stunted mental and physical development) were common in inland areas until their cause was determined to be iodine deficiency—a problem that was solved by iodized salt.

Iodine may also be an effective treatment for painful fibrocystic breast disease. (But be aware that fibrocystic changes in the breast—that is, benign lumps—are common and don't need treatment unless they cause severe pain.)

Of several types of iodine that have been tested, molecular iodine appears to be the best. (Other types have various side effects, but molecular iodine is almost impossible to get.) One study compared 23 subjects receiving molecular iodine with 33 subjects receiving a placebo. 65% of the treatment group had subjective and objective improvement; in the control group, 33% had subjective, but not objective, improvement. [Ghent]

Iron

Remember Geritol ads? In the sixties, iron was a popular remedy for "tired blood"—based on the fact that the body needs iron to carry oxygen to the cells. (Iron is still the only nutritional supplement that's regularly prescribed by doctors.)

Ironically (what else would you expect from iron?), iron supplements may also be the riskiest. There's evidence that they can increase the risk of cancer and they're the leading cause of fatal pediatric poisonings! [Litovitz]

Some people have difficulty metabolizing iron (a condition called hemochromatosis), but it can be dangerous even in normal adult men. Using data from the extensive National Health and Nutrition Examination Survey, researchers found that large stores of iron in the body increased men's risk of cancer. (The connection wasn't as clear in women.) [Stevens]

Another study found that men with high iron levels had a higher risk of colonic adenomas, which increase the risk of colon cancer. [Nelson] The iron-cancer connection is interesting because cancer patients are often anemic, a condition that physicians—with all the best intentions—used to treat with iron. But—ironically again—cancer cells need iron, so the supplements made patients' tumors grow.

Some studies have linked iron to an increased risk of cardiovascular disease, but others haven't, so more research is needed in this area. [Ascherio] Many foods that children eat are fortified with iron, and for decades it's been assumed that such supplementation is harmless, but in one study of 47 children who weren't iron-deficient, those receiving iron gained weight more slowly than those given a placebo. [Idjradinata]

Iron's not all bad: it's needed (in very small quantities) for the normal growth and development of babies—particularly premature ones—and to treat severe iron-deficiency anemia. [Lozoff] A recent study found that iron deficiency can cause restless legs syndrome in the elderly. [O'Keefe]

There are ways to manage one's iron level—exercise lowers it, and so does giving blood. [Lakka] The chance that these worthwhile activities may also reduce cancer risk is another good reason to engage in them.

Magnesium

Magnesium, a mineral that's essential for the normal functioning of muscles, nerves and bones, has long been used in conventional medicine for treating *eclampsia* (seizures associated with pregnancy). In the alternative medical community, magnesium is also well established as a treatment for heart disease, asthma and other conditions—uses that have only recently (and slowly) begun to be recognized by conventional medical practitioners.

Magnesium clearly reduces the risk of several different kinds of cardiac arrhythmias (abnormal heart rhythms). In two uncontrolled studies on a total of eighteen subjects suffering from a particular type of arrhythmia called torsades de pointes, magnesium reversed the arrhythmia in *every* subject. [Tsivoni, Perticone]

Another study looked at eighteen subjects with another kind of arrhythmia called atrial fibrillation. All the subjects were given intravenous injections of a drug called digoxin. Ten also received intravenous magnesium, while the other eight got a placebo. The fast heart rates of all the magnesium recipients went down, while the heart rates of only half the placebo recipients did. The magnesium subjects also responded almost four times faster than the placebo subjects. [Brodsky]

In 100 patients who'd just had cardiac surgery, subjects who received intravenous magnesium suffered from only half as many ventricular arrhythmias as the subjects taking a placebo. The hearts of the magnesium-treated subjects also pumped more blood after the surgery. [England]

A meta-analysis of magnesium in treating acute heart attacks found eight randomized controlled trials involving 930 subjects. The magnesium-treated group showed 49% fewer serious arrhythmias, 58% fewer cardiac arrests and 54% fewer deaths than the control group. [Horner]

As this study suggests, magnesium given after a heart attack helps people live longer. In a later, larger study of 2316 subjects four weeks after they suffered suspected heart attacks, there were 24% fewer deaths among those who had been given magnesium. [Woods 2] A long-term follow-up of the same study found that the mortality rate of magnesium-treated subjects was reduced by 16%, and the reduction for *ischemic* (oxygen-deprived) heart disease was 21%. [Woods 1]

Whether magnesium helps to lower blood pressure is debatable. Theoretically it should, since it relaxes muscle tissue, and relaxing the arteries' muscle tissue should lower blood pressure. But studies have found mixed results. Among the larger controlled trials, one found no significant effect, [THPCRG] but another trial of 91 women with mild to moderately high blood pressure found a modest but significant reduction in the magnesium subjects. [Witteman]

Another study of 71 patients found a beneficial effect of magnesium only in those who had low levels of magnesium excretion to begin with, so it may be that magnesium only helps those who are magnesium-deficient. [Lind] Low magnesium is common, however. One study of 1033 blood samples from urban primary care hospitals found that almost half were low in magnesium. [Whang]

All in all, there's enough intriguing information about magnesium and cardiovascular disease that a large, placebo-controlled trial on this topic should be done.

Magnesium may also help prevent migraine headaches, particularly those associated with the menstrual cycle. In a study of 20 women, those who took magnesium found a significant reduction in days with headaches, and in other premenstrual complaints as well. [Faccinetti] Another study of migraine patients found that the levels of magnesium within their red blood cells were lower than in patients who never got migraines. [Gallai]

A controlled trial of 38 acute asthma patients who weren't sufficiently helped by inhalers found that the airflow rates of the 19 magnesium-treated subjects improved significantly, and that fewer of them ended up being admitted to the hospital. [Skobeloff]

Magnesium is toxic in high doses, but since properly functioning kidneys can get rid of six grams of magnesium a day, it's hard to overdose on magnesium supplements (unless you have kidney problems). More than a gram a day tends to cause diarrhea, which is a good cue to cut back on your dosage.

A toxic level of magnesium in the bloodstream *can* result from abuse of magnesium-containing laxatives, intravenous overdose or kidney failure. [Higgins] The early signs are nausea, vomiting and flushing; later symptoms can include lack of reflexes and cardiac problems, including cardiac arrest.

Multivitamins

There's good evidence that multivitamin supplements or other combinations of nutrients can improve the body's immune responses and decrease rates of infection and various types of cancer. For example, in a study of rural Chinese with nutrient-deficient diets, a combination of beta-carotene, vitamin E and selenium lowered death rates by 9%, mostly due to a decrease in cancer rates. [Blot] And this was for extremely low doses of these supplements.

In another study, 96 elderly subjects got either a multivitamin or a placebo. The immune responses of those receiving the vitamins improved, and they got fewer illnesses due to infections. [Chandra]

A group of physicians who took a multivitamin decreased their incidence of cataracts by 27%. [Seddon] A study of nurses, however, found no such decrease. [Hankinson]

A group of bladder cancer patients being treated with BCG *(bacillus Calmette-Guerin)* was randomized into two sets: one got a multivitamin with the recommended daily allowance of vitamins, and the other got 40,000 IUs *(international units)* of vitamin A, 100 mg of vitamin B_6, 2000 mg of vitamin C, 400 IUs of vitamin E and 90 mg of zinc.

After a year of treatment, cancer recurred in 37% of the RDA patients but in only 9% of the group taking the high-dose vitamins. By the end of the study, recurrence was 80% in the RDA group versus 40% in the high-dose vitamin group. [Lamm]

Phytoestrogens

Chinese and Japanese women who eat traditional foods have lower breast cancer rates than those who eat a Western diet. [Adlercreutz 1] Asians eat less fat and protein (and more carbohydrates) than Westerners, and a low-fat diet is known to protect against several cancers. But there's another intriguing explanation for the lower breast cancer rate:

Both the Chinese and Japanese eat tofu, green soybeans and other soy products, which contain *phytoestrogens* (estrogen-like compounds found in plants), and the level of phytoestrogens they excrete is high. One study of Chinese women in Singapore found that the intake of soy products seemed to protect premenopausal—but not postmenopausal—women from breast cancer. [Lee]

Besides having lower breast cancer rates, Asian women complain less of hot flashes; eating phytoestrogens may serve as a form of hormone replacement therapy. [Adlercreutz 2]

Replacing meat with tofu can lower fat and calorie intake, but even when it doesn't, soy products appear to lower cholesterol levels. A number of studies have compared subjects on diets heavy on soy with subjects eating a control diet. A meta-analysis of 38 controlled trials found that consumption of soy protein reduced total cholesterol by an average of 9%, LDL by 13% and triglycerides by 10%. (There was also an insignificant increase in HDL.) [Anderson]

Soy products aren't all created equal: A recent study compared tofu, commercial soy drinks and soy-based baby formulas. Tofu had ten times as much of the phytoestrogens genistein and daidzein as the soy drinks, and infant formulas had only trace amounts. [Dwyer] Soy sauce had virtually none. [Adlercreutz 3]

Potassium

Potassium is a mineral that's necessary for normal fluid balance and nerve and muscle function. A study of 859 men and women found that 2.6 times as many people in the lowest third (those with the lowest amount of potassium in their diet) died of stroke, compared to the other two-thirds of subjects. [Khaw] Potassium may also help reduce blood pressure, but studies on this have produced inconsistent results.

Potassium can cause abnormal heart rhythms and death, and it shouldn't be taken except under the supervision of a physician who's regularly checking the level of potassium in the blood. (The amounts contained in multivitamins, however, are generally safe.)

Selenium

In areas of the country where the soil contains high levels of the antioxidant mineral selenium, cancer rates are lower. A number of case-control studies—though not all—have found that cancer patients generally have lower selenium levels than healthy people. [Combs]

Selenium also seems to have an effect on cardiovascular disease. One prospective, observational study in Denmark found that men with the lowest selenium levels in their blood were 1.7 times as likely to suffer a cardiovascular event. [Suadicani]

Selenium is toxic in doses over about 200 micrograms a day. An early sign of an overdose is a metallic taste in the mouth; later signs can include garlicky breath, fragile or black nails, dizziness and nausea.

Special diets

There's clear epidemiological evidence that diets that derive less than 20% of their calories from fat prevent cardiovascular disease, gallbladder disease, colon cancer and possibly breast cancer—but the evidence is far too extensive to review in a book of this size. Studies on the use of low-fat diets to *treat* disease, however, make up a much smaller list.

Two randomized trials of subjects with narrowing coronary arteries found that a very low-fat diet combined with exercise and stress management was able to unclog arteries that were being closed by fat deposits. [Ornish, Gould]

A diet that contains less than 20 grams of fat a day may help slow multiple sclerosis, according to a survey of 144 subjects that began in the 1950s. The subjects were advised to eat a low-fat diet, and were then followed for 34 years.

In every category of disability, those who adhered to the low-fat diet had less deterioration and lower death rates than those who didn't. Those who began the diet when they were minimally disabled derived the most benefit. This evidence isn't conclusive—since there may have been other differences between those who did and didn't follow the diet—but it should spark more research. [Swank]

Elimination or exclusion diets, in which patients avoid foods they're sensitive to, are popular in alternative medicine, but they're scorned by conventional physicians. Nevertheless, they may be effective in some cases, particularly for inflammatory bowel disease (which includes Crohn's disease and ulcerative colitis). This serious illness is typically treated with powerful drugs and, in severe cases, with surgery. Elimination diets should be the first line of treatment for these patients.

In a small, controlled study of 20 patients with Crohn's disease, ten patients received a fiber-rich diet of unrefined carbohydrates, while ten others were tested for food intolerances (often dairy and cereal products) and then placed on a diet that excluded those foods. Six months later, seven of the ten on the exclusion diet were still in remission, while none of the others were. [Jones]

In another, uncontrolled trial, an exclusion diet enabled 51 out of 77 patients to remain well for up to

51 months using the diet alone, with fewer than 10% of the patients relapsing each year. [Jones]

In a larger trial, 136 Crohn's patients were randomized into groups that got either an exclusion diet or steroids. (The foods excluded—based on patients' intolerances—were primarily cereals, dairy products and yeast.) Remissions lasted a median of 3.8 months in the steroid group and 7.5 months for those on the exclusion diet. [Riordan]

The effect of food sensitivity on rheumatoid arthritis has been known since about 1914. [Miller, Zeller] In six studies of rheumatoid arthritis patients, fasting and/or elimination diets helped symptoms in at least some patients. [Darlington]

In one study, 27 rheumatoid arthritis patients at a health farm fasted for seven to ten days, then were placed on an individually-adjusted, gluten-free vegan diet for three to five months. (A vegan diet excludes *all* foods from animal sources—not only meat but also eggs, dairy products, etc.) A control group of 26 subjects at a convalescent home ate a normal diet.

The subjects eating the special diet showed significant improvement in the number of tender joints, pain level, duration of morning stiffness, grip strength and blood tests, but this trial would be more convincing if the subjects had been randomized into the treated and control groups, and if both groups had been in the same place. [Kjeldsen-Kragh]

Conventional medicine recognizes that chocolate, caffeine, red wine and aged cheese can trigger migraines. (Oddly, caffeine taken right before an attack can occasionally help some people avert a migraine.) [Edwards] An uncontrolled trial of 60 migraine patients who tried an elimination diet suggest that other foods may do so as well. It found that 85% of patients became headache-free when ten common foods were avoided: wheat, oranges, eggs, tea and coffee, chocolate, milk, beef, corn, sugar and yeast. [Grant] (Here again, a randomized, placebo-controlled trial would have been more convincing.)

Food sensitivities are a controversial area, but there's certainly no harm in avoiding foods that seem to worsen symptoms. However, testing for food sensitivities by injecting extracts under the skin has been shown to be ineffective by a double-blind study of eighteen subjects. [Jewett]

Vitamin A

Vitamin A is a fat-soluble nutrient that's necessary for the growth and repair of cells, for the maintenance of mucous membranes, and for the formation of light-sensitive pigments in the eye. A meta-analysis of twelve controlled trials on vitamin A found that periodically giving it to malnourished children lowered their death rates 30%. For patients hospitalized with measles, death rates went down 61%. [Fawzi]

HIV-infected mothers who are deficient in vitamin A while pregnant are much more likely to transmit the virus to their babies. A survey of 338 pregnant HIV-infected women in Malawi found that the HIV transmission rate among mothers with severe vitamin A deficiency was 32%, vs. 7% among women with healthy levels of vitamin A. [Semba]

In a controlled study of 301 women with a precancerous condition called cervical dysplasia, derivatives of vitamin A called *retinoids* were applied to the cervix (the neck of the uterus). This treatment completely reversed the dysplasia in 43% of women, compared to 27% of those who used a placebo cream. However, in severe dysplasia, there was no difference between a placebo and retinoids. [Meyskens]

Vitamin A derivatives have been shown to be effective in other precancerous conditions of the skin, mouth and vocal cords. They can also cause some types of cells which indicate leukemia or pre-leukemia to revert to normal. [Lippman]

In a study of the diets of 89,494 nurses, those who ingested the most vitamin A had 16% less risk of breast cancer. When vitamin A supplements were given to those with the least of it in their diets, their risk also went down. [Hunter] In another analysis of the same data, the nurses with the most vitamin A in their diets had 39% fewer cataracts than those who had the least. [Hankinson]

Vitamin C

Vitamin C (also called *ascorbic acid* or *ascorbate)* is an antioxidant that's also involved in the synthesis of connective tissue. It strengthens blood vessel walls, neutralizes some cancer-causing substances, regulates wound healing and growth, and promotes iron absorption. There's also evidence that vitamin C may help prevent cancers of the esophagus, mouth and cervix, but it's based on studies of eating fresh fruits and vegetables that *contain* vitamin C, and there may be something else in fruits and vegetables that's protective. [Block]

There are conflicting studies about the role of vitamin C in asthma and allergy. [Bielory] There may be some short-term antihistamine effect of vitamin C, but further work must be done in this area.

In a long-term study of nurses, those who took vitamin C supplements for more than ten years had a 45% decreased incidence of cataracts. [Hankinson] High doses of vitamin C can cause diarrhea (there's a lot of individual variability as to how much). Because it increases iron absorption, it can cause problems in people who can't metabolize iron or who have iron overload problems. [Sestilli]

Vitamin C may increase blood-clotting times in patients taking the prescription anticoagulant warfarin, and in patients with a metabolic disease called G6PD deficiency, it can rupture red blood cells. In advanced cancer patients with large tumors and widespread disease, large doses of vitamin C can cause tumor hemorrhage and death. [Block]

If you take large doses of vitamin C, your body gets used to them. If you then suddenly stop taking them, a rebound scurvy can result (scurvy is the disease that results from extreme vitamin C deficiency). Rebound scurvy has also occurred in newborns whose mothers took large doses of vitamin C during pregnancy.

Conventional physicians are taught that vitamin C can cause kidney stones. A number of studies seem to show that vitamin C increases oxalate in the urine, but it turns out that this is simply because vitamin C in the urine interfered with the *test* for urinary oxalate. (Most kidney stones are composed of calcium oxalate.) Using a more modern testing method, no significant increase in urinary oxalate was found in subjects who ingested up to 10,000 mg of vitamin C a day. [Wandzilak]

Vitamin D

Vitamin D (also called *calciferol)* is an essential nutrient that helps to regulate calcium and phosphorus levels in the body. Vital to bone health, vitamin D prevents rickets in children and helps to prevent osteoporosis in adults. It may also play a role in cancer prevention, but this is controversial. [Wargovich]

Vitamin D is the only vitamin humans can synthesize, but we need sunlight to do it. Sunscreens prevent us from synthesizing vitamin D, and at least one study showed that chronic use of sunscreens decreases vitamin D levels in the blood. [Matsuoka]

This connection is important because 75% of the vitamin D people receive is from sunshine; few of us get much in our diets. Although the milk we buy is fortified with D, many—if not most—adults can't or won't drink milk, and other dairy products like yogurt, cheese and ice cream usually aren't fortified.

Older adults are at particular risk of vitamin D deficiency, perhaps they're less able to absorb it through their intestines. [Ebiling] Fish—especially eel, herring, mackerel and salmon—are an excellent source of vitamin D, and of course it's available in capsules as well. [Garland]

Vitamin D affects calcium absorption and a massive overdose of it (40,000 IU a day for 1–4 months) can raise the level of calcium in the blood to the poiint where it causes nausea, vomiting, weakness, headache, bone pain, osteoporosis or calcifications in heart and blood vessels. [EM]

Vitamin E

Vitamin E (also called *tocopherol)* is an antioxidant that maintains the integrity of cell membranes, and is needed to synthesize DNA. A very interesting pair of studies published recently looked at vitamin E's effect on coronary heart disease.

The Health Professionals Follow-Up Study of 39,910 male physicians found that those who took a supplement of at least 100 IUs of vitamin E daily for at least two years had 37% less coronary disease than those who didn't. [Rimm] Women in the Nurse's Health Trial who took vitamin E supplements for at least two years had 41% less major coronary disease. [Stampfer 1] (Although 100 IUs is a modest amount for supplementation, it's extremely difficult to get that much from food alone.)

Vitamin E may decrease the aggregation of platelets (a component of the blood that causes clotting). A recent study found that in subjects with *transient ischemic attacks* (also called *TIAs* or *ministrokes),* aspirin and vitamin E were more effective than aspirin alone in reducing both illness and death. [Steiner] Vitamin E also appears to enhance immune response in premature infants and in the elderly. [Meydani]

Patients receiving chemotherapy often develop ulcers in the mouth or other parts of the digestive tract. In a controlled trial of eighteen cancer patients, six out of nine receiving vitamin E oil experienced resolution of their ulcers within five days, compared to only one out of nine subjects receiving a placebo. [Wadleigh]

In a study conducted in four regions of the United States, people who had at some time regularly consumed vitamin E supplements had a lower rate of oral and throat cancer than those who hadn't. [Grudley]

Zinc

Zinc is a mineral important in fertility, wound healing, taste, the synthesis of DNA and other proteins, and various other biochemical processes.

In a small, controlled study of 24 patients with rheumatoid arthritis, those who took zinc supplements experienced less joint swelling and morning stiffness, and the amount of time they could walk without discomfort increased. [Simkin] While two other studies found no effect of zinc on rheumatoid arthritis, [Mattingley, Rasker] a study of 24 subjects with psoriatic arthritis also found zinc to be beneficial. [Clemmensen]

Although there have been reports that taking zinc gluconate lozenges can shorten the duration of the common cold, [Eby, Godfrey] most studies haven't found this to be true. [Douglas, Smith, Farr] Still, different formulations may have different effects, and it's possible that flavoring agents like citric acid and sorbitol may inactivate the zinc. [Zarembo]

Zinc is toxic in large quantities, and can cause nausea, vomiting, diarrhea and abdominal pain. Even small quantities over an extended length of time can deplete copper in the body. So if zinc supplementation continues for more than a month, it's wise to consider copper supplementation as well.

EXERCISE

Those who think they have not time for bodily exercise will sooner or later have to find time for illness.
Edward Stanley, Earl of Derby (1826–93) [Stanley]

Exercise may be the most important single thing you can do to prevent disease and promote your own health. Not only does it lower rates of serious conditions like heart attack and diabetes, it's even an effective treatment for a variety of common ailments, from depression to bed-wetting.

A study of 16,936 male Harvard alumni found that those who expended 2000 or more calories (technically, *kilocalories*—but they're commonly called simply *calories)* a week had death rates a quarter to a third lower than less active men. [Paffenbarger] Similar results were found in the MRFIT (Multiple Risk Factor Intervention Trial), a study of 12,138 men. At a seven year follow-up, the death rate for those who had engaged in moderate leisure-time physical activity was only 70% that of those with low leisure-time physical activity. [Leon]

Fortunately, exercise is something that everyone can afford to do. While some of us may feel that the only fun exercise is sex or dancing, the fact is that everyone can find some form of exercise they can tolerate and do on a regular basis. (For information on a gentle Chinese form of exercise called T'ai Chi, see the chapter on miscellaneous therapies.) Climb, jog, jump, lift, walk, swim, sway or squeeze—being active improves both physical and mental health.

You don't have to work out daily, or even three times a week; getting sweaty even once a week has significant health benefits. But if you've been lying on a couch since the 1960s, lifting nothing heavier than a can of beer, don't leap up suddenly and run a marathon. Sudden heavy physical exertion can *trigger* a heart attack in those who are usually sedentary. However, as you'll see below, *regular* exercise protects against this risk. [Mittleman, Willich]

Heart attack and stroke

Numerous studies show that regular exercise can protect against cardiovascular disease. [Salonen, Curfman, Garcia-Palmieri, Hambrecht] In a group of 3043 male railroad workers, those that expended the least energy died from coronary heart disease at a rate 40% higher than that of the workers who expended the most energy. [Slattery]

A recent study of 1453 Finnish men aged 42 to 60 found that those who reported exercising more than two hours weekly had a 60% reduction in their risk of heart attack, compared to the least active men. [Lakka] A Norwegian study found that the fittest men reduced their heart attack risk by 46% and that a high level of fitness was associated with lower mortality from all causes. [Sandvik]

A meta-analysis of exercise and heart disease found that being sedentary almost doubled the risk of developing coronary heart disease, and the studies that were the strongest methodologically showed a larger benefit than those that were less well-designed. [Berlin]

95

Physical activity was also found to protect against stroke in men in a study of about 4000 men and women (although there was no protective effect for women). The benefit was highest in older men and medium levels of exercise were just as effective as high ones. [Kiely]

Diabetes

Regular exercise can also decrease the incidence of adult-onset diabetes. A study of male alumni of the University of Pennsylvania tracked the number of calories they burned during various activities (the range was from 500 to 3500 calories a week). For each 500 calories spent in activity, the risk of diabetes dropped 6%. [Helmrich]

In a study of male physicians in the Physicians Health Trial, doctors who exercised only once a week experienced a 23% drop in incidence of diabetes. Those who exercised five or more times a week reduced their risk by 42%. [Manson]

Cancer

People who engage in daily physical activity also have a lower cancer risk than inactive people. One study using data from the National Health and Nutrition Examination Survey showed that inactive men were almost twice as likely as very active men to develop cancer. The rate for inactive women was about 1.3 times that of very active women. (Interestingly, this particular study didn't find a strong association between reduced cancer risk and recreational exercise; the connection was with normal daily activity.) [Albanes]

A case-control study matched 545 women diagnosed with breast cancer before age 40 with similar women without breast cancer. Women who had exercised an average of 3.8 hours or more a week since puberty had a risk of breast cancer only 42% that of inactive women. [Bernstein]

Depression

Exercise not only prevents depression, but it's been shown to be an effective *treatment* for depression as well. An epidemiological study found that increased participation in exercise, sports and physical activities is associated with improved psychological well-being, including decreased symptoms of depression, anxiety and malaise. [Ross]

Several comparative studies have also been done. One found that running was as effective as psychotherapy. [Griest] Another that compared running to meditation and relaxation therapy and to group psychotherapy in 74 patients found that all three reduced the subjects' level of depression. [Klein]

Another study divided 43 women into three groups: subjects assigned strenuous exercise, those assigned relaxation exercises and a control group that received no treatment. It found that subjects in the aerobic exercise group experienced reliably greater decreases in depression than did subjects in the other two groups. [McCann]

Aging

Exercise can have dramatic benefits even very late in life. In a small but remarkable study, ten frail nursing

97

home residents, who ranged in age from 86 to 96, undertook eight weeks of high-intensity resistance training. They increased their strength 174%, sped up their gait 48% and pumped up their thighs 9%. The increase in their lower-extremity strength ranged from 61% to 374%. [Fiatarone 1]

In a larger, controlled trial by the same investigator, 100 frail nursing home residents were divided into four groups. The first group was given high-intensity progressive resistance training; the second group got a multinutrient supplement that contained fat, carbohydrates, protein, vitamins and minerals; the third group got both; and the fourth group got neither.

After ten weeks, muscle strength increased by 113% in the exercisers, compared to 3% in the nonexercisers. Gait velocity increased 12% in the exercisers and declined by 1% in the nonexercisers. Stair-climbing ability increased 29% in the exercisers vs. 3.6% in the nonexercisers. The multinutrient supplement on its own didn't reduce muscle weakness or physical frailty. [Fiatarone 2]

Another study of 49 nursing home residents aged 64 to 91 compared twice-weekly exercise sessions with twice-weekly sessions in which the subjects talked with the investigators (as a control, so both groups were getting the same amount of attention). After seven months, the exercise group did significantly better than the talking group on grip strength, bending from the waist (trying to touch their toes), how long it took to get out of a chair, activities of daily living and self-ratings of depression. [McMurdo]

Exercise can help postmenopausal women increase their bone mass (loss of which increases the likelihood and severity of broken-bone injuries). In one study, 48 healthy postmenopausal women were randomized to an aerobic exercise group, a group doing both aerobic and strengthening exercises, or a control group. After one year, the women in both exercise groups gained bone mass and had higher levels of fitness than the controls, who lost bone mass. [Chow]

Urinary incontinence and impotence

Urinary incontinence is a common problem, for adults as well as for children. It's more frequent among women than men—half of the elderly female population suffers from it. The most common form is stress incontinence, which causes urine loss when coughing, sneezing or lifting heavy objects (in its most severe form, it can cause urine loss in any upright position).

The standard treatment for stress incontinence is surgery, which can overcompensate and make urinating difficult. A much less traumatic treatment is something called the Kegel exercise; it's been shown to help not only incontinence and bed-wetting, but also impotence. (For how to do it, see the end of this section.)

A study of fifty female patients compared surgery to the Kegel exercise and found that although surgery was superior, 42% of the Kegeling patients were so much improved that they didn't want surgery. [Klarskov] In another study of 36 women who were taught the Kegel exercise, 36% considered their stress incontinence cured, 19% thought it was substantially improved and 44% felt their problem was unchanged.

Urinary flow studies showed that the problem was actually improved in all women who thought it was. [Elia]

A study of 79 children who experienced daytime incontinence (nearly two-thirds of whom also experienced bed-wetting) found that after two hours of Kegel training, 60% were completely cured and 14% had a partial reduction. [Schneider]

And in a group of men with impotence due to leaking veins, the Kegel exercise was almost as good as surgery in restoring erections. 42% of patients who finished the training program were satisfied with the outcome and refused surgery. [Claes]

One great thing about the Kegel exercise is that you can do it anywhere, anytime, without anyone noticing a thing. To learn how to Kegel, try stopping your urine midstream; the Kegel exercise is nothing more than contracting the muscles that do that. (It isn't a good idea to keep doing that when urinating; it's just for learning purposes. Once you know how to do it, you can Kegel any time.) The usual prescription is 60–80 Kegels a day, both quick flicks and longer contractions (held for a maximum of 5–10 seconds).

Not everyone can learn to Kegel with verbal instruction alone, so Kegeling aids exist. Various forms of vaginal balloons are used, sometimes in combination with biofeedback. Weighted vaginal cones are also used. You start by retaining the lightest cone for a set amount of time, then gradually increase the weights. [Brubaker] (Going out in public with the weights inside you is a wonderful motivation for retaining them.)

HERBS

Anyone who's lain awake after an evening cappucino, or experienced the stimulating effect of prune juice, knows that plants—and products made from them—can have a powerful impact on our bodies. When plants are used for such effects, rather than as food, they're called *herbs*—or, more precisely, *medicinal herbs* (to distinguish them from *culinary herbs,* which are used to season food). In the strictest definition, only soft-stemmed plants are herbs, but I'm using the term here in the more common, broader sense of all useful plants. (Herbs are also discussed in the *aromatherapy* and *essential oils* sections of the last chapter.)

Herbs have been used medicinally for thousands of years, all over the globe; in fact, virtually no human culture has ever been discovered that doesn't use them. The use of herbs isn't even restricted to the human species. Chimpanzees swallow without chewing a medicinal herb called aspilia that kills parasites and bacteria. (They clearly don't like the taste, since they often grimace when they swallow it.) [Bower]

Herbal medicine may utilize a whole plant or just the bark, fruit, stem, root or seed. Herbs can be purchased fresh or dried, and in pills, capsules and *tinctures* (preserved in alcohol, glycerine or some other liquid).

Although about a quarter of our pharmaceutical drugs are derived from herbs, [Foster] physicians have a strange double standard about them, believing that they're simultaneously clinically ineffective and dangerous. In other words, they consider herbs to be all side effect and no benefit.

On the other side is an equally absurd viewpoint: that herbs are incapable of causing harm because they're "natural." While an argument can be made that herbal medications may be gentler than their pharmaceutical cousins because they're less concentrated, and because their effects may be buffered by other compounds in the plant, herbs contain a staggering variety of active ingredients that can have profound effects, both good and bad, on humans.

A *standardized extract* is one that's guaranteed to contain a specific amount of a particular active ingredient. (Obviously, extracts can only be standardized when the active ingredient is known—or believed to be known.) Standardized extracts are useful because the concentration of active ingredients can vary greatly in different parts of a plant—or even within the same part of the plant in different seasons, soils or climates.

Some herbs are more dangerous than the drugs derived from them. Digitalis is a good example. Used to strengthen the contractions of a weak heart, it was originally isolated from foxglove *(Digitalis purpurea)*. The amount of active ingredient in foxglove varies substantially, a serious matter when a therapeutic dose is uncomfortably close to a fatal dose (as it is in this case). Because it's more consistent, pharmaceutical digitalis is safer than foxglove.

Some herbs are harmless even in large quantities, but others should be used only under the guidance of an herbalist or other knowledgeable professional. Possible adverse effects of herbs are mentioned throughout this chapter, and there's an extended discussion on the subject at the end of the chapter.

Several common painkillers owe their origins to herbs. The chemical basis for aspirin was originally discovered in white willow bark *(Salix alba)*. Aspirin was later synthesized from the same chemical in meadowsweet *(Spiraea ulmaria)*, from which it derives the *spir* in its name.

The opium poppy gives us narcotics. A related poppy provides the seeds that adorn bagels and that flavor cakes, strudel and the triangular Jewish pastries called *homentashen*. Indulging in such treats can cost you your job if your company screens for drugs in your urine, because the poppy seeds used in baking can trigger a laboratory diagnosis of narcotics use!

Herbs are the basis for many other kinds of medicines as well. A key player in the sexual revolution—the birth control pill—was derived from the Mexican yam *(Dioscorea villosa)*. Vincristine and vinblastine, used in cancer treatment, come from the Madagascar periwinkle *(Catharanthus roseus)*. Taxol, used to treat breast and ovarian cancer, was discovered in the Pacific yew *(Taxus)*.

(When taxol's effects were first documented, there was a great deal of concern over potential destruction of an uncommon plant. However, it was soon learned that taxol can also be found abundantly in the ornamental yew, a popular hedging bush.)

Similar or identical compounds are often found in different plants, even when they're not closely related. For example, the unmistakable flavor of licorice *(Glycyrrhiza glabra)* is also found in fennel *(Foeniculum vulgare)* and anise *(Pimpinella anisum)*, which are in a completely different family. All three plants have distinct medicinal uses.

These three aren't the only culinary herbs that are also used medicinally; other examples include garlic, onions, ginger, parsley, sage, rosemary and thyme (the last four are used musically as well). But be aware that just because certain plants are used as food doesn't necessarily mean they're the safest ones; nutmeg, for example, is harmless when grated onto eggnog, but it's toxic in large quantities (more than one whole nutmeg).

Many Western herbalists use *simples* (preparations of a single herb), but in Chinese and in ayurvedic medicine, many herbs are usually blended together. Small quantities of toxic herbs may be included to stimulate the immune system, and sometimes animal or mineral substances are added as well. Like cooking, the blending of herbal mixtures is a high art, in which various ingredients augment or modulate each other.

Chinese herbal mixtures have been found to be effective in both children and adults with atopic eczema. [Sheehan 1 & 2] Another Chinese formulation was also effective in the treatment of children with acute bronchiolitis (an inflammation of the lung, potentially serious in babies) that's caused by respiratory syncytial virus. In a single-blind trial, 96 children were randomly given antibiotics, Chinese herbs or a combination of both. The children who got the herbs, with or without antibiotics, got over their symptoms—fever, cough and wheezing—earlier. [Kong] (Ayurvedic herbs and herbal mixtures are discussed in the chapter on ayurveda.)

Below you'll find a small sampling of individual medicinal herbs that have been proven to be effective for certain ailments. I've listed them in alphabetical order and, where applicable, I've put their scientific names in parentheses after the common ones. (Unless otherwise noted, a capitalized scientific name indicates a genus and a lowercase name indicates a species.)

Bromelain

Bromelain, an enzyme derived from the stems of pineapple plants *(Ananas comosus)* may help reduce swelling and inflammation. In a double-blind trial of 160 women who'd received a mediolateral episiotomy (a particularly painful, diagonal variety of that incision that's rarely used nowadays), those who took bromelain had less swelling and pain than those who took a placebo. [Zatuchni]

Chili peppers *(Capsicum)*

The fact that topically applied chili peppers can decrease pain has enabled this herb to cross over into conventional medicine; the active component, capsaicin, has been incorporated into a cream used on arthritic joints. (It sometimes causes burning or stinging, but this usually disappears after a few doses.) One double-blind, controlled study of 21 patients found that capsaicin cream reduced tenderness and pain of osteoarthritis patients by 40%, but it had no effect on patients with rheumatoid arthritis. [McCarthy]

Besides arthritis, topical capsaicin is useful for diabetic neuropathy (nerve pain, tingling or numbness, usually in the legs, caused by diabetes). One study of

252 patients with this ailment found that 70% of patients treated with the capsaicin cream reported pain improvement to their physicians, compared to 53% of those on the placebo. The intensity of pain was also lessened in the capsaicin group. [CSG]

Of 45 patients treated with capsaicin or a placebo for fibromyalgia (a pain syndrome characterized by exquisitely tender "trigger points"), those receiving capsaicin reported less tenderness at their trigger points. A significant increase in grip strength was also noted. [McCarty]

Post-herpetic neuralgia is a condition in which patients suffer severe pain or itching long after an attack of herpes zoster—commonly known as shingles—has resolved. In an uncontrolled study, capsaicin cream was reported to provide good to excellent pain relief in more than half of the 23 patients who completed the study. [Watson 2] A later, controlled trial confirmed these results: of 32 elderly patients with post-herpetic neuralgia, almost 80% of the capsaicin-treated patients experienced some relief from their pain within six weeks. [Bernstein]

A small, controlled study of 23 patients found that capsaicin cream is also helpful in postmastectomy pain syndrome (nerve pain that persists after the operation). Five of thirteen patients receiving the capsaicin cream reported good to excellent results, compared to one out of ten patients in the placebo group. [Watson 1]

Capsaicin has even been used in a surgical procedure for loin pain/hematuria syndrome, a condition in which patients have kidney pain and blood in the urine. Under general anesthesia, capsaicin was introduced into the hollow part of the kidney through a catheter (tube). While the treatment appeared to help the original pain, it produced severe bladder pain and the feeling of having been kicked in the kidneys. [Bultitude] Although these effects were temporary, it's not at all clear that substituting one pain for another makes much sense.

Cranberries *(Vaccinium macrocarpon)*

Women, especially those who use diaphragms, are more prone to urinary tract infections than are men, and are sometimes placed on daily (or precoital) doses of antibiotics. Cranberry juice might work just as well. It acidifies the urine, and also seems to make it more difficult for bacteria to stick to the bladder wall. [Sobota]

In one study, 153 elderly women drank 300 ml a day of cranberry juice or a placebo juice matched for taste, appearance and vitamin C content. White blood cells and bacteria (both signs of infection) appeared in the urine of those who got the placebo drink twice as often as in the urine of those who drank the cranberry juice. [Avorn]

Researchers in Israel tested a number of fruit juices to see how well they inhibited the adhesive ability of *E. coli,* the most common cause of urinary tract infections; they found that only cranberry and blueberry juices were beneficial. [Ofek] It makes sense that both these juices would have a similar effect, since they're relatives: both berries belong to the genus *Vaccinium.*

Echinacea (Echinacea augustifolia or purpurea)

Echinacea, an herb that boosts the immune system, is commonly used in Europe—especially in Germany, where more than 300 preparations of it are available. Most of the literature on echinacea is in German, but there's increasing interest in this herb in the US.

A review of 26 controlled clinical trials (18 randomized, 11 double-blind) looked at groups treated with pure echinacea extracts or mixtures containing the herb. Nineteen trials studied whether the preparation prevented or cured infections (most commonly colds or flu), four studied the reduction of side effects of cancer therapies, and three studied whether echinacea affected indicators of immune function.

The primary authors of the studies that were reviewed claim positive results for 30 of the 34 groups. Although the evidence does point to echinacea having a positive effect on the immune system, the authors of the review note that most of the trials were of poor methodological quality and don't provide enough information to make clear recommendations about how much of which preparation to use, and under what circumstances. [Melchart]

Evening primrose oil (Oenothera biennis)

The evening primrose is a roadside weed that particularly favors railroad tracks. It has beautiful yellow flowers that open in the evening and then stay open throughout the next day. [Weiss]

Evening primrose oil—which is usually abbreviated EPO—is high in the essential fatty acids (EFAs) linoleic and gammalinolenic acid (which are also found in black currant seed and borage seed oil). EFAs were also used in the 1930s and 1940s for eczema, but they aren't generally used for that purpose today. However, there have been several, more recent studies of EPO that show it may be an important treatment for this condition.

A trial of 414 patients with breast pain—both cyclic (related to the menstrual cycle) and noncyclic (constant)—found that EPO was as effective as the prescription drug bromocriptine, but not as effective as the prescription drug danazol. However, EPO had fewer side effects than either drug. [Gately]

In one study of 99 patients with atopic (allergic) eczema, subjects in the high-dose groups—who received eight to twelve capsules a day for adults, and four capsules a day for children—had less itching, scaling and general severity. Lower doses helped only itching, with adults responding better than children. [Wright] Another study of seventeen children and fifteen adults with eczema found that EPO was more effective than a placebo (as reported both by the patients and by physicians assessing the condition). [Lovell] A third study also found a beneficial effect. [Schalin-Karrila]

One rheumatoid arthritis study gave sixteen patients EPO, fifteen EPO and fish oil, and eighteen a placebo for a year. 73% of the EPO group, 80% of the EPO/fish oil group and 33% of the placebo group were able to stop taking painkillers, or reduce how many they were taking. (A few patients in the treated groups experienced nausea, diarrhea or headache.) [Belch]

Another study of 37 rheumatoid arthritis patients found that, in patients who completed 24 weeks of treatment, gammalinolenic acid from borage seed oil decreased tenderness and swelling, and improved pain, the ability to perform tasks and global assessments by physicians. [Leventhal] However, a third study that used olive oil as the placebo found no difference between it and EPO (neither was very effective). [Brzeski]

Feverfew (Tanacetum parthenium)

Several good trials show that the herb feverfew prevents migraine headaches. In one study, subjects who ate feverfew leaves daily to prevent migraines were randomly given either dried feverfew leaves or a placebo. Those who received the placebo had a significant increase in the frequency and severity of headaches, nausea and vomiting, while those in the feverfew group showed no change in the incidence of their migraines. This study was small (only seventeen subjects) and only tells us about the effect of withdrawing feverfew from regular users. [Johnson 1]

In a larger, crossover study, 72 migraine patients were given either one capsule of dried feverfew or a placebo daily for four months, then were crossed over for four more months. During the time they were treated with feverfew, patients had fewer migraines, less severe attacks and less vomiting, although the duration of individual attacks remained the same. [Murphy]

Many migraine sufferers grow feverfew and eat a few leaves every day, but this can cause mouth ulcers, loss of taste and swelling of the mouth, lips or tongue in sensitive people. [Awang] Taking the herb in capsules should reduce these effects, but it won't completely eliminate them.

Garlic *(Allium sativum)* **and onion** *(Allium cepa)*

Members of the *Allium* family, which includes garlic and onion, have several different effects that work together to help the cardiovascular system. For example, garlic appears to have some antioxidant effects that could help protect arteries. [Phelps]

A meta-analysis of five good trials that looked at the effect of garlic on cholesterol found that the equivalent of one-half to one clove of garlic daily lowered serum cholesterol about 9% in the groups of patients studied. [Warshafsky]

In a trial of healthy volunteers and patients with coronary heart disease (CHD), 88 participants were given either garlic or a placebo for six to eight months. Garlic decreased total cholesterol 20% in the healthy volunteers and 18% in those with CHD; triglycerides and LDL (low-density lipoprotein—the "bad" cholesterol) also fell, while HDL (high-density lipoprotein—the "good" cholesterol) rose. [Bordia 2]

Another double-blind study of 40 patients with high cholesterol found that after four months, total cholesterol fell 21% in the group taking garlic, compared to a 3% reduction in the control group. Triglycerides also fell 24% in the garlic-treated group vs. a 5% reduction in the control group. [Vorberg]

A more recent, double-blind, placebo-controlled study found a more modest effect: garlic tablets reduced LDL cholesterol 11% and total cholesterol about 6%, while cholesterol levels went down 1% in the placebo group. [Jain]

Garlic and onions also thin the blood. The clumping together of platelets is an important mechanism for stanching the blood flow from a cut finger, but it can cause fatal damage when clumps form within blood vessels. Two studies found that alliums inhibit the clumping of platelets in human blood, and another laboratory study found that a specific component of garlic called *allicin* had the same effect. [Bordia 3, Kiesewetter, Mayeux]

Studies have been mixed on whether garlic helps hypertension (high blood pressure), but in one double-blind trial of 47 patients with mild hypertension, diastolic blood pressure dropped from 102 to 89 after twelve weeks (the placebo group showed no significant change). Cholesterol and triglycerides also dropped in the garlic-treated group. [Auer]

Lipids in the blood rise within a few hours of eating fat, but this effect is reduced by garlic or onion. [Bordia 1] To my mind, this constitutes an argument for infusing one's entire butter supply with garlic. Actually, when cows eat a lot of garlic or onions, their milk takes on the scent, so maybe dairies could start selling garlic butter prepared right inside the cows. But I digress.

Alliums may help prevent gastrointestinal cancer as well as heart disease. In mice, garlic inhibits the development of colon cancer [Wargovich] and inhibits promotion of skin tumors. [Nishino] In humans, the higher the allium intake, the lower the stomach cancer rates. In the part of Georgia known for Vidalia onions, the stomach cancer mortality rate among whites is only a third the national level and half the state level. [You]

Bacteria may play a role in stomach cancer, so the antibacterial properties of alliums may be part of the explanation. Garlic and onion have been shown to kill several types of bacteria, including several nasty gastrointestinal denizens. [Johnson 2] Given the emergence of multiple antibiotic-resistant bacteria in both hospitals and communities, the development of allium antibiotics should certainly be pursued.

Ginger *(Zingiber officinale)*

Ginger clearly helps nausea and vomiting due to various causes, but conflicting results on motion sickness indicate that more research needs to be done in that area. (I'm not volunteering.)

In a double-blind study comparing ginger, the antinausea drug metoclopramide (Reglan) and a placebo, ginger was as effective as metoclopramide in preventing the nausea and vomiting that frequently occurs after surgery. [Bone] And a placebo-controlled laboratory study of eight volunteers found ginger more effective than the placebo in controlling induced dizziness, one of the symptoms of motion sickness. [Grontved 2]

Ginger has also been shown to be superior to Dramamine (dimenhydrinate) for preventing laboratory-induced motion sickness. In one study, 36 undergraduates ingested Dramamine, capsules of powdered ginger or capsules of a placebo herb. They were then blindfolded and placed in a tilted, rotating chair for six minutes—or until they threw up, requested freedom or experienced three triplings in the magnitude of nausea. None of the subjects in the placebo or Dramamine group could stay in the chair for six minutes, but half of those in the ginger group could. [Mowrey]

Ginger's usefulness for real-life motion sickness is less clear. A placebo-controlled trial of 80 naval cadets in heavy seas found that ginger reduced the number of vomiting episodes and cold sweats, but didn't significantly reduce nausea or dizziness. [Grontved 1] (A single dose of one gram was used, and it's possible that a higher dose would have had a more beneficial effect.) A recent study of 28 volunteers found ginger ineffective when compared to scopolamine and a placebo. [Stewart]

In a double-blind, crossover trial of 30 women with severe morning sickness, each woman received ginger capsules or a placebo for four days, then nothing for two days, then ginger or the placebo (whichever she hadn't taken before) for four days. 70% of the women preferred the ginger, which reduced both the degree of nausea and the number of attacks of vomiting. [Fischer-Rasmussen]

Ginkgo *(Ginkgo biloba)*
An ancient tree whose fan-shaped leaves turn a brilliant yellow in autumn, the ginkgo has no living relatives; it's the only member of its family and genus. The fresh fruit—or "nut," as it's incorrectly called—is delicious, and is a prized food in China. In the US, however, the planting of female (fruit-bearing) trees is avoided. This is because rotting ginkgo fruit smells

like dog poop (the fresh fruit is odorless).

Ginkgo appears to have a direct effect on blood vessels, helping increase blood flow without changing blood pressure. It's widely used for circulatory problems in France and in Germany, where it's one of the most frequently prescribed drugs. Fifteen controlled trials all showed that ginkgo can help with intermittent claudication (pain in the legs on walking, due to inadequate blood flow)—although only two of these trials were deemed to be of acceptable quality. [Kleijnen 2]

Since it increases flow in small blood vessels, ginkgo can relieve memory problems and confusion that are caused by cerebral insufficiency (diminished blood flow to the brain). In a meta-analysis of about 40 studies done on this topic, seven of the eight best placebo-controlled trials showed that ginkgo was more effective than a placebo for a variety of patient complaints, including memory and concentration problems, headaches, depression and dizziness. [Kleijnen 1] In a recent double-blind study of 40 patients with early Alzheimer's disease, those who received 240 mg of ginkgo daily scored better than controls on memory, attention and social functioning. [Hofferberth]

Ginkgo may also help one type of impotence. In 60 men with impotence caused by arterial flow problems, ginkgo improved blood flow within eight weeks; after six months, half of the men had regained potency. Although this wasn't a placebo-controlled trial, and was apparently published only as an abstract, the results were interesting—especially considering that these were men whom conventional treatment hadn't been able to help. [Sikora]

Ginkgo may also have antioxidant properties, but there's been far less work in this area. [Dumont]

Ginseng (Panax)

Ginseng is widely used in Asia as a tonic. The Asian variety *(P. ginseng)* and the American variety *(P. quinquefolius)* are used for different purposes in Chinese medicine. American ginseng is highly prized in China, and much of the ginseng used in China is actually grown in the US. So-called Siberian ginseng *(Eleutherococcus senticosus)* isn't in the same genus as Asian and American ginseng, although it does have medicinal effects of its own.

An epidemiological study in Korea found a lower overall rate of cancer, and decreased rates of lung, liver, oral and throat cancers in particular, in people who consumed red or white ginseng extract or powder. However, neither fresh ginseng nor white ginseng tea showed this effect. [Yun]

This study isn't sufficient on its own, however, and more research needs to be done—especially since ginseng doesn't appear to be a completely benign herb. It can cause high blood pressure and there have been case reports of abnormal bleeding in women who are past menopause (an estrogenic effect). [Punnonen, Hopkins, Greenspan]

Licorice (Glycyrrhiza glabra)

Many children know that black licorice, not red, is the real one. But if the black licorice is from the US, chances are that it's actually flavored with anise. Most imported licorice candy is made from real licorice, however, and we do use real licorice in laxatives, chewing tobacco and "naturally sweet" teas (licorice is many times sweeter than sugar).

Licorice is an important anti-inflammatory herb, widely used in Chinese medicine. It also affects the metabolism of the steroid hormone cortisol. This can cause quite serious adverse effects—long-term users of licorice may suffer from edema (swelling caused by fluid retention), high blood pressure and low potassium. [Farese, Epstein] There was even a case of cardiac arrest (which the patient fortunately survived). [Bannister] These effects appear to be due to glycyrrhizinic acid, which is one of several active ingredients in licorice.

Numerous studies have shown licorice and licorice compounds to be very effective in treating stomach and intestinal ulcers, and removing the glycyrrhizinic acid doesn't seem to affect this ability (whose mode of action appears to be promotion of the secretion of protective mucus). [Doll, Turpie, Tewari, Cliff, Amure] In one study of more than 500 patients with confirmed intestinal ulcers, deglycyrrhizinated licorice (DGL) was compared with antacids and cimetidine (Tagamet); patients in all three groups healed equally well. [Kassir] DGL also works as a maintenance treatment to help prevent recurrences, [Morgan] and reduces the incidence of gastrointestinal bleeding caused by aspirin. [Rees]

(We know now that most ulcers are caused by a bacterium called *Helicobacter* and should be treated with antibiotics.)

Milk thistle (Silybum marianum)

Milk thistle protects the liver, but most of the extensive literature on this effect is in German. In one of the few studies published in English, rats given toxins from the deadliest mushroom known—*Amanita phalloides,* the "poison deathcap" or "deadly angel"—were protected by a component of the milk thistle called silybin. [Tuchweber]

Preparations of milk thistle are used in Germany today to treat human victims of amanita poisoning. That's a relatively rare problem, of course, but other forms of liver disease—such as hepatitis and cirrhosis—are quite common.

In one double-blind study of people admitted to a Finnish military hospital for liver disease, 47 patients who received silymarin (a combination of different active ingredients) had a greater decrease in two liver enzyme tests than the 50 controls. Some patients had before-and-after liver biopsies and, here again, treated patients showed more improvement than controls. [Salmi] The problem with this study is that the only thing the subjects had in common was increased liver enzymes, which can be caused by many different conditions—including infection, alcoholism and several medications, including acetaminophen (Tylenol).

In a better study of 170 patients with cirrhosis (a scarring of the liver often, but not always, associated with alcoholism), subjects who received silymarin were less likely to die than those who received a placebo. Silymarin seemed more effective in subjects whose cirrhosis was less severe, or was alcohol-induced. [Ferenci]

More research on silymarin must be done to determine which liver diseases it helps most. If it's useful in treating infectious hepatitis, tens of thousands of lives could be saved annually.

Onion *(see Garlic)*

Pineapple enzyme *(see Bromelain)*

St. Johnswort *(Hypericum perforatum)*
Eight trials found the herb St. Johnswort (a common roadside weed in much of the US) superior to a placebo for treating depression. Three trials comparing it to standard antidepressants found both treatments equally effective, but subjects receiving St. Johnswort had fewer side effects. [Ernst] But be aware that ingestion of this herb can cause photosensitivity (which means you get sunburned more easily).

Saw palmetto *(Serenoa repens)*
Although not commonly used for food nowadays, the fruit of the dwarf palm, or saw palmetto, used to be an important food source for Southeastern Native American tribes. An extract of saw palmetto has been shown to improve the symptoms of prostate enlargement. A double-blind study of 110 patients in France found that urinary flow rate improved by 50%, and the number of nighttime trips to the bathroom decreased significantly. [Champault]

Saw palmetto inhibits an enzyme which converts one type of testosterone to another, a process thought to be important in the development of both enlargement of the prostate and prostate cancer. A prescription drug called finasteride (Proscar), which treats prostate enlargement by inhibiting the same enzyme, is being tested in a federally-funded trial of 18,000 men, in order to see whether it prevents prostate cancer.

Finasteride isn't a particularly dangerous drug, but it causes impotence or loss of libido in a small percentage of men who use it, and it can cause birth defects in children of women who handle the pills or are exposed to semen of a man using the drug. Saw palmetto may have the same beneficial effects as Proscar with fewer side effects—in fact, saw palmetto has a reputation among herbalists as an aphrodisiac!

Sweet wormwood *(Artemisia annua)*
Long an herbal remedy for parasites, including those that cause malaria, sweet wormwood (also called *sweet Annie,* or *quinghao* in Chinese) is staging a comeback—especially now that there are drug-resistant strains of malaria. Several studies show its effectiveness. [Jiang, Li]

A trial of artemisinin (the active ingredient of sweet wormwood) in 638 malaria patients in Vietnam showed a dramatic success rate—parasites in the blood decreased more than 98% within 24 hours and were completely gone in 48 hours. [Sy] Recurrence of symptoms is high with short-term use of artemisinin, but it works faster than known drugs.

Sweet wormwood is sometimes used to flavor vermouth. There's no apparent toxicity with short-term use of it, but another species of wormwood, *Artemisia absinthium,* is the primary flavoring ingredient of absinthe. That liqueur felled many a drinker in the nineteenth century, and has since been made illegal virtually everywhere.

Valerian *(Valeriana officinalis* and other species)
Herbalists consider valerian root a potent anti-anxiety drug and sedative. Here again, much of the literature on this is in German, but two double-blind trials in English also found that valerian preparations induce sleep.

In one study, a preparation containing *Valeriana officinalis* with other ingredients was compared to an extract containing only valerian; both were tested against a placebo. Both valerian preparations helped subjects fall asleep more quickly, and enhanced the quality of sleep. [Leathwood]

In the other study, 27 patients with sleep difficulties received two pills; they took one the first night and the other the second. Both pills contained hops and lemon balm, but one pill contained only 4 mg of valerian while the other contained a full 400 mg dose. (Both hops and lemon balm are mild sedatives; valerian is considered to be much stronger.) 78% of the subjects found the full-dose valerian preparation more effective; 15% liked the low-dose valerian; and 7% had no preference. [Lindahl]

Adverse effects of herbs
The effects of herbs—like those of pharmaceutical drugs—vary according to the age, weight, genetics, sex and biochemistry of each individual. Herbs can also

interact with drugs, and the two should only be used at the same time under the supervision of a knowledgeable health care practitioner.

Despite that, adverse effects caused by herbs are rare. 80% of food-related complaints reported to the Food and Drug Administration relate to aspartame (Nutrasweet) and 15% to sulfites, which are used as preservatives. [Folkenberg] Relatively few plant poisonings are reported, and they're almost exclusively due to consumption of toxic ornamental plants, not herbs. [McCaleb]

For example, the oleander bush *(Nerium oleander)* is so poisonous that a hot dog roasted over a fire on an oleander twig may contain enough poison to kill an adult. The sickly-sweet, gelatinous berries of the ornamental yew *(Taxus)* are edible, but they might make for an anxious meal: the seeds inside the fruit contain an alkaloid so poisonous that four are enough to kill a grown man. (Birds eat the fruit with impunity because they don't crack the seeds, which pass through their digestive tracts intact.)

Despite dangerous ornamental plants like these, plant poisonings are seldom serious—98% of those reported to US poison control centers between 1985 and 1990 resulted in minor or no toxicity. [Jacobsen] Ten fatalities were reported during the same period, the majority of which were due to poison hemlock *(Conium maculatum)*—which has a superficial resemblance to parsley—or water hemlock *(Cicuta maculata* or *douglasii)*. Neither plant is used medicinally—although hemlock, of course, is what was used to execute Socrates.

122

In 1989, plant poisonings resulted in one fatality, compared to 414 deaths caused by antidepressants, analgesics, sedatives and heart drugs. [McCaleb] Still, herbs should be treated with respect. Even correctly identified ones may have both mild and severe side effects. [Huxtable 2] For example, ma huang *(Ephedra sinica)* can increase blood pressure and heart rate, which can be dangerous in someone with cardiovascular disease (especially hypertension).

At the same time, just because a plant contains a toxin doesn't mean it's toxic. Cabbage, for instance, contains a substance that can cause goiter, but unless one is subsisting on coleslaw and sauerkraut, no harm results from eating a lot of cabbage. Poison is always a question of dose.

The most dangerous compounds in medicinal herbs are the pyrrolizidine alkaloids, which can lead to liver problems and death, especially in children. Pyrrolizidines occur in comfrey *(Symphytum)*, borage *(Borago officinalis)*, coltsfoot *(Tussilago farfara)* and species of *Crotalaria* and *Senecio*, all of which are (or have been) used in herb teas—especially in Jamaica, Africa, South and Central America. Liver toxicity has also been associated with chaparral *(Larrea divaricata)*, [Katz, Gordon] germander *(Teucrium chamaedrys)* [Larrey] and a Chinese medicine called *jin bu huan*. [Woolf]

Food plants can also cause illness. Potatoes, tomatoes and eggplant all belong to the *Solanaceae* (nightshade) family, and they all contain *solanine*, the poison that's found in their close relative, the deadly nightshade. All parts of the potato plant *(Solanum tuberosum)* are poisonous except for the edible tuber, and even that can be poisonous when green or sprouted. [Arena]

Peruvians, however, regularly eat a type of potato with a high solanine content, and apparently suffer no ill effects from that. While consumption of the black nightshade *(Solanum nigrum)* can be fatal to some people, it's used as a vegetable by the Hmong of Laos and the Luo-speaking tribes of Kenya. [Fackelmann]

Why would the same plant poison some populations and not others? There are several possible explanations. A lifelong diet of black nightshade may confer the ability to metabolize the poison, or perhaps methods of preparation reduce the solanine to harmless levels (Kenyans boil this bitter herb in several changes of water—although the Hmong, apparently, don't).

A number of common foods must be processed to be safe. Uncooked beans contain a substance that causes blood cells to stick together. [Jaffé] The root of the cassava *(Manihot esculenta)* is poisonous when fresh, but quite edible after it's been processed into tapioca. [Conn]

Some plants are edible only at certain times of the year. Many a youngster has been warned away from unripe fruit because of the threat of a stomachache, but eating certain other plants out of season will cause much worse effects than a stomachache. The stems of pokeweed *(Phytolacca americana)* are edible in the early spring but become poisonous as they mature and redden. The ackee fruit *(Blighia sapida)* is harmless when ripe but can block the synthesis of sugars in the liver when unripe, causing dangerously low blood sugar and even death (this used to be a common plant-associated poisoning in Jamaica). [Huxtable 1]

So—you have to know what you're doing. Herbs can make a valuable contribution to preventive health care as well as to the treatment of disease, but they need to be properly identified (misidentification is more common than one might imagine), prepared in a way that maintains potency, labelled as to their indications and contraindications, and used in correct dosages.

HOMEOPATHY

Homeopathy is a comprehensive system of medicine with a wide following in India and continental Europe and a smaller but dedicated clientele in the United States (1% of all US adults). However, it's based on concepts that make conventional doctors cringe. For example: its remedies are chosen for their potential to *reproduce* the patient's symptoms; the more these remedies are diluted, the *stronger* they get; and symptoms are given more importance than diseases.

Samuel Hahnemann, the German physician who originated homeopathy in the early 1800s, is said to have been curious about how cinchona bark (the source of quinine) worked to cure malaria. Experimenting on himself, he discovered that cinchona *produced* the symptoms of malaria. From this he developed the idea that symptoms were an expression of the body's resistance to a disease, and that cinchona kindled this resistance. [Vithoulkas 1]

Eventually Hahnemann evolved *the doctrine of similars,* or *like cures like.* (The name *homeopathy* comes from the Greek *homoios,* "similar" and *pathos,* "suffering.") [Stedman's] Hundreds of animal, vegetable, and mineral substances were "proved" (tested) on healthy people, whose symptoms were painstakingly recorded. A substance that caused a symptom in a healthy person was then labelled a *remedy* and used to treat the same symptom in a sick person.

Full doses, however, often made the patient's symptoms much worse before effecting a cure, so Hahnemann experimented with diluting remedies in order to find the minimum dose necessary to cure a condition without worsening it. He found that remedies maintained their potency even when they were diluted repeatedly. In fact—surprisingly—remedies became *more* effective the more they were diluted.

(Homeopaths call this *potentization by dilution.* If *potentization* has sent you scurrying to your dictionary, don't bother. Homeopaths use lots of specialized jargon and this is an example. It simply means *potentiation*—i.e. making more powerful.)

For example, a quantity of an herb might be diluted in ten times as much water and vigorously shaken (or *succussed*—another example of homeopathic jargon) 40 to 100 times. A small portion of the resulting solution will then be itself diluted 10-to-1 in water, and this procedure will be repeated 30 times, with the last dilution always done in alcohol. [Vithoulkas 2]

The end result is a 30X solution *(X* being the Roman numeral for 10, 30X indicates thirty 10-to-1 dilutions). Although it's very unlikely that even a single molecule of the original herb will remain in a 30X solution, homeopaths successfully use these preparations as remedies for various ailments.

Homeopathic remedies sold in most US health food stores fall into the lowest potency range (that is, the *least* diluted), usually going no higher than 30C *(C* being the Roman numeral for 100, 30C indicates thirty 100-to-1 dilutions).

How does potentization by dilution work? Homeopaths claim that, even if no molecules remain from the original substance, a "message" somehow remains imprinted on the diluting liquid. This message or "ghost" can't be detected by laboratory analysis—its effect is evident only in the response of the patients to whom it's given.

In a homeopathic consultation, the practitioner doesn't try to diagnose a particular disease, but rather tries to build up as detailed a picture as possible of both the patient's symptoms and his or her personal characteristics. The choice of remedy is greatly influenced by factors such as the individual's general attitude toward life, preferences in food and surroundings, and sleep patterns.

In homeopathy, symptoms are all-important. If, for example, a rash develops during treatment, it is viewed as an indication that the disease is working its way out of the body. [Coulter]

The only side effect of homeopathic remedies may be a transient—but sometimes dramatic—worsening of symptoms. This "aggravation" of the symptoms (as homeopaths called it) can be as serious as a severe asthma attack or pancreatitis. Nevertheless, homeopaths generally consider aggravations to be favorable signs, as it shows that the remedy is a good match for the illness.

The modern homeopath draws on a massive database, now sometimes computerized, that links remedies with particular constellations of symptoms and/or with temperamental profiles. Since Hahnemann's time, the "proving" (testing) of remedies on healthy volunteers has been a central element of homeopathic research, and has generated a homeopathic pharmacopeia of about 2000 items. [Jacobs 2] Since 1938, all listed remedies have been recognized as drugs by US statute.

Homeopathic practice isn't uniform throughout the world. In India, South America, and the United Kingdom, the predominant mode is classical homeopathy, which looks for a precise match between a patient's symptoms—both physical and temperamental—and a single remedy. In France and Germany, it's more common for a mixture of remedies to be prescribed. [Boyd] This approach is known as *polypharmacy.* Both types of practice can be found in the United States.

US demand for homeopathic products languished in the decades during and after World War II, but it has increased dramatically since the 1970s (along with burgeoning interest in all forms of alternative medicine). Some homeopathic companies saw their sales soar by up to a thousand percent in just a few years in the late seventies and early eighties. [FDA]

Today, mixed remedies are widely available over the counter for flu, vaginal yeast infections and other common maladies. One example of these pathology-based—as opposed to symptom-based—homeopathic remedies, in which the same treatment is given to everyone with a particular ailment, is the popular flu remedy Oscillococcinum *(uh-SIL-uh-KOK-sin-um).* It's made of the heart and liver of a duck that are soaked for forty days before being processed.

In 1806, Hahnemann wrote: "No substance is poisonous when taken in its correct dose." [Hahnemann] Although homeopathic preparations sometimes utilize toxic, inedible or unpalatable ingredients, the multiple dilutions ensure that remedies won't cause any serious adverse effects.

Homeopathy and conventional medicine

According to the medical historian Harris Coulter, the formation of the American Institute of Homeopathy in 1844 was the direct cause of the founding two years later of the American Medical Association. The AMA maintained a hostile stand toward homeopathy throughout the remainder of the nineteenth century, a period during which homeopaths enjoyed their greatest popularity. (Statistics for 1890 show that there were approximately 14,000 homeopaths in the United States, about one-sixth the number of conventional physicians.) [Coulter]

Between 1850 and 1880, regular physicians were sanctioned even for associating with homeopaths. In the late 1870s, a New York doctor was expelled from his medical society for purchasing milk sugar (used in making homeopathic preparations) at a homeopathic pharmacy. A physician in Norwalk, Connecticut, was similarly punished when he came under suspicion of having consulted with a homeopath—who happened to be his wife! (The decision was later thrown out for lack of evidence.) [Starr] This staunch opposition eventually took its toll: by the 1930s, homeopathy was drifting toward extinction. [Coulter]

Hostility toward the profession has been extremely slow to abate. As recently as the early seventies, a medical dictionary defined homeopathy as a "cult" and stated that "the real value of homeopathy was to demonstrate the healing powers of nature and the therapeutic virtue of placebos." [Stedman's]

Hahnemann called conventional physicians *allopaths* (from the Greek *allo,* which means "other" or "different"). While homeopathy seeks a medicine that matches the patient's symptoms, allopathy looks for a medicine that opposes them. Allopathic medicines can, among other things, kill bacteria, reduce fever, suppress coughs and stop diarrhea. But rather than working in concert with a patient's natural defense mechanisms, they often contradict and override those defenses.

Whereas homeopathy takes all its cues from the patient's descriptions of symptoms, modern allopathic medicine regards symptoms as simply the subjective feelings of those who are unqualified to judge their own condition. Symptoms are diagnostic distractions. Diseases, all caused by mechanical or physiological changes, must be seen, touched or biopsied to be believed. The doctor, in other words, must be able to validate the patient's experience. Illnesses without visual or palpable signs are dismissed as unworthy of attention.

Not surprisingly, homeopathy's central concept of potentization by dilution is the one that draws the most scorn from allopaths. Looking into a medicine that contains no detectable agent, they see only a potential placebo.

Their skepticism is an understandable response to a system that contradicts accepted scientific principles. And it isn't helped by the fact that some homeopaths scoff at the usefulness of scientific trials, maintaining that homeopathy is so different from allopathic medicine that it can't be tested by conventional methods. What's more, they typically believe that nothing is incurable—it's just a question of finding the right remedy. So, in a flawlessly circular argument, they say that if a remedy doesn't work, it merely indicates that the homeopath chose the wrong one.

More reasonable advocates argue that science hasn't yet evolved to the point at which the mechanism of homeopathy can be demonstrated, and they remind skeptics that just because you don't know *how* something works doesn't mean it doesn't work. (Aspirin was used for almost a century before medical science pinned down its actual mode of action.) And, as you'll soon see, scientific trials have been done that demonstrate that homeopathy *does* work.

Despite their radical differences, allopathy and homeopathy do share a number of concepts—for example, the notion of using a small amount of a disease-causing substance to combat disease. Conventional allergy desensitization shots use small doses of bee venom or other allergen to coax the irritable immune system into ignoring the stimulus. Vaccination uses killed or crippled germs to rehearse the body for a battle against the real thing.

Another shared concept is "appropriate dose." While homeopathy uses infinitesimal doses, much of standard medical treatment depends on the use of dangerous drugs in safe quantities. On the first day of my pharmacology course in medical school, a professor scrawled on the blackboard, "Drugs are poisons," to remind us that the drugs we would be prescribing were potent and had to be used judiciously.

Even the concept of a medicine that can cause the same symptoms it is meant to cure isn't unknown in allopathy. Lidocaine, which can provoke irregular heartbeats, is also used to treat them. Radiation is known to cause cancer, yet cancer is commonly treated with radiotherapy. Although the popular drug Prozac (fluoxetine) is highly successful in treating depression, in some cases it worsens the problem. And while decongestants can have a magical effect on a stuffy head, too much of them can increase congestion (the so-called "rebound phenomenon").

Perhaps a day will come when a truce is called in the ongoing skirmishes between homeopathy and allopathy, and these two distinct forms of medicine will acknowledge a much larger base of common understanding. Meanwhile, there's a pressing need for large-scale scientific studies of homeopathic treatment, so that homeopathy's theoretical and clinical arguments can rest, not on a belief in "ghosts," but on the quantified evidence of flesh and blood.

Effects on animals

As already noted, there are those who dismiss the apparent benefits of homeopathic treatment among human patients as pure placebo effect. But this argument is difficult to extend to animals, and in Europe, veterinary diseases are often treated homeopathically.

One controlled—though not double-blind—study of a herd of sows that was suffering a high miscarriage rate found that ten sows treated with homeopathic caulophyllum had only half the stillbirths of ten controls. Subsequently, the entire herd of 130 was given the same remedy and the piglet mortality rate dropped from 20% to 2.6%. When the treatment was withdrawn, mortality rose to almost 15%, and when it was reinstated, the rate fell back to 1.9%. [Day]

Effects on human cells

In 1988, the respected biological science journal *Nature* caused a major stir—one might even call it a panic—in the scientific community when it published an article on the effect of homeopathy on cellular activity. A study by an international team of researchers found that a human white blood cell called a basophil, when isolated from human blood and exposed to a homeopathic dilution of immunoglobulin E antiserum, released histamine. [Davenas] Although it was known that normal doses of immunoglobulin E stimulate histamine release, the discovery that the homeopathic version achieved the same result stunned the mainstream scientific audience, because there was no reason to believe that the homeopathic solution contained even a single molecule of the antibody.

Nature placed an unprecedented statement on the last page of the article, observing that "there is no physical basis for such an activity." The journal also made clear that it had published the article only on the condition that the findings be independently investigated by its own team of experts.

This team of experts was a motley crew composed of a professional magician, a journalist and a scientific fraud expert. After spending a week in the French laboratory of Drs. Davenas and Benveniste, the team devised a blind experiment, the results of which failed to support the published results. [Maddox] An enraged— in fact, almost incoherent—response by Dr. Benveniste pointed out that the conclusions were based on a single experiment using two samples of blood in poor condition and that the results had been interpreted by overextended researchers under stressful circumstances. [Benveniste]

The dispute over the *Nature* article remains unresolved. However, the important issue isn't whether human cells respond to homeopathy, but whether human beings do.

Respiratory ailments
In a randomized, double-blind study of 144 Scottish hay fever sufferers, a homeopathic mixture of grass pollens was given to half of the participants and a placebo to the other half. The patients who received homeopathic treatment showed a clear reduction in symptoms, halving their use of antihistamines. The placebo group, on the other hand, showed no significant change. When the results were corrected for varying pollen counts in different parts of Glasgow, the contrast between the two groups was even more pronounced. [Reilly 2]

Actually, this study tested neither classical homeopathy nor homeopathic polypharmacy, but a related approach called *isopathy*, which uses the exact substance that causes the disease. (Other homeopathic remedies are based on substances that reproduce the *symptoms*, regardless of what actually causes the disease.)

In another double-blind trial by the same investigator, fourteen patients with allergic asthma were given homeopathic immunotherapy using whatever substances they were allergic to, while fourteen similar patients were given a placebo. (All these subjects were also receiving conventional therapy.) The "well-being" score of the homeopathic group rose beyond that of the control group after one week and the difference persisted for up to eight weeks. [Reilly 1]

However, a randomized, placebo-controlled study of 175 Dutch children with recurrent upper-respiratory infections concluded that the group receiving individualized homeopathic therapies didn't differ significantly from the control group. [de Lange de Klerk]

Various ailments

A Scottish double-blind study tested classical homeopathy in 46 patients with rheumatoid arthritis and found that, after three months, the patients who received individualized homeopathic treatments of anti-inflammatory drugs showed improvement in pain, joint tenderness, stiffness, and grip strength. [Gipson]

A double-blind, crossover study of fibrositis patients for whom homeopathic *Rhus toxicodendron* was prescribed found that treatment with this remedy resulted in a 25% reduction in the number of *trigger points* (places on the body that are exquisitely tender to the touch). [Fisher]

A double-blind, placebo-controlled study of 60 migraine sufferers gave one dose of an individualized homeopathic remedy every two weeks for eight weeks. The placebo group dropped from 9.9 attacks per month to 7.9—an effect that remained at follow-up examinations two months after the study ended. In the treated group, the incidence of migraines dropped from 10 to 3 per month, and at the two-month follow-up, the number had dropped to 1.8. The intensity of attacks also decreased significantly in the treated group. [Brigo]

In a double-blind, controlled study of acute diarrhea in 81 Nicaraguan children between the ages of six months and five years, patients who received individualized homeopathic remedies had a statistically significant decrease in the duration of diarrhea and in the number of stools per day after 72 hours of treatment, as compared to the placebo group. [Jacobs 1]

A homeopathic preparation for influenza (remember the marinated duck innards?) was tested in 237 patients in France; another 241 received a placebo. 17% of those treated with the remedy recovered within 48 hours of treatment vs. 10% of those who received the placebo. [Ferley]

Meta-analysis

Three physicians in the Netherlands looked at all controlled human trials of homeopathy that had been published anywhere in the world up to 1990. Of 105 trials, 14 tested classical homeopathic prescriptions of single remedies, 26 tested combination treatments, 58 gave the same homeopathic remedy to a group of patients with comparable conventional diagnoses, and 9 tested isopathy. The researchers found that 75% of interpretable trials showed a positive result.

The authors point out that many of the trials weren't very well designed, but note that "there is no reason to believe that the influence of publication bias, data massage, bad methodology, and so on is much less in conventional medicine, and the financial interests for regular pharmaceuticals companies are many times greater." [Kleijnen]

HYPNOSIS AND IMAGERY

Apart from poisoning by stealth, there is no form of therapy from which the effects of suggestion can be entirely eliminated.   *George Day* [Day]

About 5–10% of the population are very susceptible to hypnosis, 25–30% are minimally so, and everyone else falls in between. (Some people are so responsive that they can undergo major surgery with hypnosis as their only anesthesia.) [Hilgard]

Despite the movie stereotype of evil hypnotists making people in trances do things against their will, hypnosis works best when there's a great deal of trust involved. (That's one reason self-hypnosis can be so effective. In fact, some hypnotists claim that "all hypnosis is self-hypnosis.") [Torem]

There are two contemporary schools of hypnosis. Traditional hypnosis works with the "enhanced suggestibility" that occurs in deep, formal trances. In the approach pioneered by Milton Erickson, however, hypnosis is "an altered state of mind" and behavior is affected by the everyday trances that we all experience.

For Ericksonians, hypnosis is everywhere. Daydreaming, watching a sunset, losing track of time while absorbed in a book or a conversation, missing an exit as you watch the white lines on the highway slip monotonously under the wheels of your car—all can be thought of as types of hypnosis (so can advertising, which may explain your credit card bills).

139

Imagery is often used in hypnosis, and has been shown to increase blood sugar and stomach secretions, inhibit gastrointestinal activity and alter skin temperature. [Shiekh] In *guided imagery*, the technique most often used with relaxation, biofeedback, hypnosis, meditation or behavioral therapy, specific images—as well as sounds, smells, etc.—are suggested.

A study of 55 mothers of premature infants found that the 30 who listened to a twenty-minute relaxation/imagery audiotape produced 63% more breast milk than the 25 who didn't. The more frequently a mother listened to the tape, the more milk she was able to produce. [Feher]

Imagery can also be used on its own, and not just to treat disease. In one survey of elite athletes, 99% reported using imagery techniques to enhance performance. [Orlick]

The history of hypnosis

In 1778, an Austrian physician named Franz Mesmer moved to Paris and began treating patients by putting them into a bath-like structure lined with iron filings and magnets. The success of this approach attracted people from all over Europe, but it was less popular with his colleagues, who pressured the French Academy to appoint, in 1784, a commission to investigate him.

The blue-ribbon commission—which included Benjamin Franklin, the chemist Lavoisier and Dr. Guillotin, inventor of the guillotine—devised what may have been the first controlled trial of a therapy ever performed. Because Mesmer said that some of his patients were so sensitive that they would have seizures if they touched trees that had been magnetized, the commission had certain trees in an orchard magnetized.

Unfortunately for Mesmer, his patients reacted to trees they were told had been magnetized—or that they'd seen being magnetized—rather than to ones that actually *had* been. Mesmer was denounced as a fraud, but his success with patients—which was, it turned out, based on his rapport with them, rather than on magnets—laid the groundwork for modern hypnosis. [Erickson]

Interest in Mesmerism was revived by (among others) the English surgeon James Esdaile. He performed hundreds of major operations in India on hypnotized patients and wrote *Mesmerism in India,* a book still considered a classic.

Another English doctor, James Braid, developed the eye-fixation, watch-the-swinging-watch technique and coined the term *hypnosis* (from *hypnos,* the Greek word for sleep). When he realized that trances weren't sleep, Braid tried to change the term to the unpronounceable *monoeidism (*meaning concentration on one idea), but *hypnosis* is the one that stuck.

Hypnosis didn't become firmly ensconced as a valuable therapeutic tool until around World War I, when a German psychoanalyst, Ernst Simmel, combined it with psychodynamic techniques. Today, the effectiveness of hypnosis for certain medical purposes is widely accepted, but it's been underutilized for chronic, difficult-to-treat conditions like asthma, fibromyalgia, irritable bowel syndrome, weight control and pain—despite the convincing studies described below.

Ichthyosis

One of the most famous cases of medical treatment by hypnosis involved a 16-year-old boy with ichthyosis, or fishskin disease, a condition in which hard scales form on the skin. (This patient was covered with a black, hard coating over his entire body except for his chest, neck and face.) Several operations to transfer normal chest skin to his palms failed—the transplanted skin grew as rigid as the removed skin.

Under hypnosis, a suggestion was made that the boy's left arm would clear. Five days later, the black casing began to fall off, and in ten days it was gone. Through further hypnosis, other parts of the body also improved tremendously. [Mason] Dramatic case reports like this are, of course, never enough to go on by themselves, but a number of controlled trials of hypnosis also show positive results.

Asthma

In one trial, twelve subjects who were highly susceptible to hypnosis had improved symptoms, decreased use of medications and dramatically decreased response to methacholine (a substance that usually worsens asthma), as compared both to the seventeen controls and to ten other subjects who also were hypnotized but whose susceptibility to it was low. [Ewer]

A controlled trial of 252 asthmatics found that progressive relaxation therapy and hypnosis both reduced symptoms, but hypnosis was more effective. Independent assessment found 59% of the hypnosis group "much better," compared to 43% of the relax-

ation group (a statistically significant difference). [RRC]
Another controlled trial of 62 patients found that hypnosis reduced both the use of drugs and the number of
days on which wheezing occurred. [Maher-Loughnan]

Nausea

In an uncontrolled study of 138 pregnant patients with
severe vomiting (not just morning sickness, but all day
long) that wasn't helped by medication, a brief hypnosis
treatment led to improvement in 88% of the subjects.
(Both group and individual hypnosis treatment worked,
but group treatment was much more effective.) [Fuchs]

Up to a quarter of patients undergoing chemotherapy develop such an averse reaction that they get nauseated or start throwing up even before the drugs are
administered. There are many cases in which this problem—called anticipatory vomiting—has been relieved by
hypnosis, as has been confirmed by two studies. [Redd 2]

In one small study, three cancer patients were
treated with hypnosis before some sessions of
chemotherapy but not before others, and three others
were treated before all their sessions. None of the
patients vomited after hypnosis, but all vomited when
they didn't get it. [Redd 1]

In another trial of 60 patients, hypnosis was also
shown to significantly reduce anticipatory vomiting.
(This study was notable both for appearing in the pres-
tigious New England Journal of Medicine and for
assiduously avoiding the term hypnosis, calling it
instead "systematic desensitization" or "behavioral
therapy.") [Morrow]

Irritable bowel syndrome

Irritable bowel syndrome (often abbreviated *IBS*) is a common disorder that can cause cycles of diarrhea and constipation. In an uncontrolled study, 33 patients with IBS that didn't respond to medical treatment received four sessions of group or individual hypnotherapy (all were taught self-hypnosis techniques as well). After seven weeks, a third of the patients were symptom-free, 27% had improved, and the remaining 39% got no benefit. [Harvey]

One researcher did two related studies on IBS. The first, a randomized, controlled trial of 30 subjects, compared hypnotherapy to psychotherapy. The hypnotherapy helped patients dramatically, but psychotherapy was far less effective. [Whorwell 2]

In a second, follow-up study of 15 treated patients from the first study plus 35 others, patients younger than 50 with classic IBS symptoms had a 100% response rate to hypnosis, while the rate for patients over 50 with classic symptoms was only 25%. (For subjects with atypical symptoms, the rate was 43%— regardless of their age.) [Whorwell 1]

By 1989, this researcher had followed 250 patients (including those in the two previous studies) and found that hypnosis helped up to 80% of them. [Whorwell 3] Since there's no effective conventional treatment for IBS, hypnosis should be the treatment of choice for severe cases of this condition.

Pain

Another condition with no successful conventional treatment is fibromyalgia, a syndrome of muscular aching and stiffness with multiple tender points. In a controlled study of 40 fibromyalgia patients, those who were hypnotized reported less pain and less fatigue on awakening than those who received physical therapy. [Haanen]

For the pain of breast cancer, hypnosis has been found more effective than a support group or no treatment. [Spiegel] Another study of 67 cancer patients undergoing bone marrow transplants compared hypnosis, cognitive behavioral skills, contact with a psychologist, and no treatment. Hypnosis proved to be effective in reducing oral pain (a common side-effect of chemotherapy), but nothing seemed to help nausea, vomiting or the need to use painkillers. [Syrjala]

In 49 children and adolescents with cancer, hypnosis with imagery proved more effective than nonhypnotic behavioral techniques (deep breathing, distraction and practice sessions) in reducing pain and the anxiety connected with spinal taps and bone marrow biopsies. [Zeltzer]

Stopping smoking

The use of hypnosis is more accepted by the medical community for smoking cessation than for other conditions, but the evidence of its efficacy is controversial. Hypnosis and smoking studies have been criticized for relying on patients' own reporting of how often they smoke (substance abusers are notoriously inaccurate about how much of a substance they're abusing) and for the lack of long-term follow-up.

In a review of seventeen studies, the percentages of people treated by hypnosis who still weren't smoking after six months ranged wildly from 4% to 88%. However, in programs that offered several hours of treatment, intense interpersonal interaction, individualized suggestions and follow-up treatment, success rates were above 50%. [Holroyd]

Weight control

Hypnosis has been found to be effective in weight loss. In a controlled study, obese patients received either hypnosis, hypnosis plus an audiotape, or just an equivalent amount of attention. Both hypnosis groups lost an average of about seventeen pounds in six months, while the control group gained half a pound. [Cochrane]

In another study, 45 obese subjects trying to lose 9 kg (20 lbs) in 90 days were divided into three groups. All were shown graphs of their daily weights, encouraged to try to keep them under a declining line, and told to eat less. Subjects who additionally received hypnosis with specific food aversion suggestions lost an average of 6.4 kg. Those who got the hypnosis but not the food aversion suggestions lost 3.4 kg. Those who received no hypnosis lost only 1.3 kg. [Barabasz]

Highly hypnotizable subjects did better in this study, as well as in another uncontrolled one, where the most highly hypnotizable subjects lost more than 20 lbs. [Anderson]

MASSAGE AND BODYWORK

Conventional medicine once involved more physical contact; in fact, when the stethoscope was first introduced, its opponents argued that it distanced physicians from patients, who were used to having the doctor lay his ear on their chest. Modern medicine continues this distancing trend: we physicians probe our patients with instruments, needle them for lab tests, send them into dark tunnels for CAT scans and sometimes monitor them on video screens, rather than watching them directly.

Everyone needs to be touched. But in American culture, there aren't many socially acceptable, nonsexual forms of touch besides dancing, having one's hair or nails done, the hugs and slaps athletes indulge in after a victory...and bodywork. *(Bodywork* is a general term that covers massage and many other kinds of therapy, all of which have in common touching and/or moving the body.)

According to a Harvard telephone survey, 7% of Americans used massage therapy in 1990—but probably 100% of us rubbed out a leg cramp or a bonked elbow. The rubbing instinct is a good one: if done correctly, it can loosen a cramp, or speed healing of an injured area by bringing more blood to it.

However obvious the benefits of massage and bodywork may be to those who've received them, they aren't well documented in available literature, and it's not clear which effects are due to actual massage techniques and which to mere attention and touch. More answers may come to light upon translation of a large

147

body of massage therapy literature that's said to exist in Europe—especially East Germany—and in the former Soviet Union.

Types of massage and bodywork

Massage was a part of many ancient cultures, including China, India, Persia, Arabia and Greece. But of the 80 different methods of massage therapy recognized today, only about 20 are over 20 years old. [Brennan]

In the US, there are currently four major categories of bodywork. The best-known is European massage, of which Swedish is the most popular. It involves long gliding strokes, kneading and friction.

Deep tissue techniques make up a second major category. The most famous of these is *structural integration* or *rolfing,* which is described toward the end of this chapter. Other variations include Aston Patterning and Hellerwork.

A third category includes *pressure-point* techniques like *reflexology* and *acupressure* (pressing with the fingers on acupuncture points—for more about what those are, see the acupuncture chapter). *Shiatsu* is a popular Japanese form of acupressure.

Polarity therapy, *Reiki, jin shin jyutsu* and *jin shin do* are similar to pressure-point techniques but are specifically concerned with moving energy through the body in order to balance it. *Therapeutic touch* is a related approach that's described at the end of this chapter.

A fourth category, *movement integration*, includes the Feldenkrais and Alexander techniques, both of which teach better ways to move one's body to reduce stress. (There's more about Feldenkrais below.)

Other popular kinds of bodywork combine different techniques. For example, traditional Chinese massage combines rubbing strokes with localized pinching, tapping, twisting and pressing motions.

Premature babies

Several studies suggest that touch may facilitate premature babies' growth and development. While most infants get touched more than enough by doting relatives, the only times little preemies in plastic incubators may be handled is to have needles poked into their veins. (Interestingly, even painful touch has some positive effect, but pleasant touch is more beneficial.)

A small study compared six preterm babies who were stroked and had their arms and legs flexed for an hour a day with six infants who received only normal nursery care. The stroked babies ate more, gained weight faster, and weighed more at the end of the study than those who received only normal care. [White]

In the best premature-baby study, 20 infants who were stroked for three ten-minute periods a day for ten days gained an average of 47% more weight per day, were more active and alert, showed more mature behaviors, and left the hospital an average of six days earlier than 20 others in the intensive care unit. [Field 2]

In another ten-day study of 30 cocaine-exposed premature newborns, the ones who got three fifteen-minute massages a day gained an average of 28% more weight daily than the untreated babies—without eating more food. The massaged group also had fewer medical complications and showed more mature motor skills. [Wheeden]

Less massage appears to be less effective. In another ten-day controlled study of 40 premature infants, the treated babies got just one fifteen-minute massage per day. They started to eat more on days six to ten, but didn't gain significantly more weight than the untreated group. [Rausch]

Anxiety

In a five-day study of child and adolescent psychiatric patients, daily 30-minute back massage reduced anxiety and depression more effectively than a relaxing videotape. [Field 1] Another, uncontrolled study of cancer patients found that therapeutic massage reduced pain perception by 60% and anxiety by 24%. [Ferrell-Torry]

Back massage also reduced anxiety in elderly institutionalized subjects, but not by a significantly greater amount than conversation. [Fraser] This study points up the problem of inadequately controlled studies—merely giving attention to people can make them feel better, so that effect must be controlled for.

Edema

Massage also reduces *edema* (swelling) due to blocked lymphatic vessels. In one study of 60 post-mastectomy subjects with arm edema, getting lymphatic massages three times a week for four weeks resulted in a significant reduction in edema that lasted at least three months.

A pneumatic device used for six hours a day was also effective when it exerted constant pressure, but not when it applied variable pressure. [Zanolla] (Although many hospitals use such devices, most people would certainly prefer getting a massage to wearing a device for six hours a day.)

Pain

In one uncontrolled study, 21 of 26 patients with muscle pain gained some relief from massage. [Danneskiold-Samsoe] In thirteen subjects with soft tissue injuries, a few minutes of friction massage relieved pain for periods ranging from 20 seconds to 48 hours (the mean was 26 hours). [de Bruijn] An uncontrolled study of fourteen patients with inflammatory bowel disease found that massage, combined with deep-breathing exercises, increased the ability to sleep and the feeling of control over pain. [Joachim]

In a pair of studies on dental pain, using ice to massage acupuncture points on the hand and arm reduced dental pain by half. Lightly massaging the same areas with a wooden ball was far less effective. [Melzack 1 & 2] In another study, ice massage relieved lower back pain as effectively as a TENS machine (a device that uses electrical stimulation). [Melzack 3]

Frozen shoulder

In a study of 235 subjects with frozen shoulder (i.e. limited mobility of the shoulder joint), all 205 who were treated with gradual stretching and massage showed improvement, and 71% recovered completely. Of the other 30—who had their joints forcefully manipulated while under anesthesia—only a third improved and only 10% recovered completely. [Li]

Respiratory function

Massaging patients who have chronic bronchitis—especially tapping their back and chest—helps remove mucus, thus improving breathing. [Pham] Called chest physical therapy, this type of massage is also often used for hospitalized pneumonia patients.

Other effects

It's generally accepted that massage relaxes muscles and relieves muscle spasms and cramps, but there aren't many published studies in this area. One study notes that the ability to bend forward from the waist improves after massage. [Nordschow]

According to several studies, slow, stroking massage has various temporary effects on heart rate and blood pressure. (What these effects are seems to vary from study to study—or even from person to person.) [Bauer, Yates] Massage of the lymphatic system increases urine output and changes the levels of neurohormones excreted in the urine. [Kurz] Massage also appears to thin the blood for some reason. [Ernst]

Patients on bedrest are prone to develop blood clots in their legs, which can be dislodged and travel to the lungs, heart or brain. [Hill] To prevent this from happening, such patients normally get injections of blood-thinning medication (which can cause bruising or bleeding) twice a day, or wear pressurized leggings.

It's possible that regular massage of the legs could improve the circulation there enough to prevent blood clots from developing in the first place (but these leg massages would probably have to happen several times a day). Future research should investigate this possibility.

Today, massage therapists avoid bony prominences (knees, elbows, vertebrae or anywhere else bones are close to the skin). But in the past, nurses would commonly massage these areas, thinking they were lowering the risk of bedsores. In fact, the practice can actually increase bedsores. [Dyson, Olson]

Rolfing

Structural integration or *rolfing*—named after its inventor, Dr. Ida Rolf—deals with the *fascia*, tough sheaths that cover all the muscles in our bodies. According to Rolf, the fascia can get stuck together and hold the body out of alignment. In a series of ten, hour-long, deep, often painful manipulations, the fascia are separated from one another. This brings the head, shoulders, thorax, pelvis and legs into more perfect alignment, and lets one stand erect with less muscular effort.

Rolfing the pelvic area has been shown to decrease the angle of pelvises that are tilted anteriorly (that is, where the top of the pelvis is tipped forward and the bottom backward). [Cottingham] In a five-week study of 48 students, those who were rolfed scored lower on tests of anxiety than those who performed a series of exercises and movements. [Weinberg]

153

In a study of ten cerebral palsy patients, rolfing allowed mildly impaired subjects to walk faster, with longer and more even strides. But moderately impaired subjects walked only slightly faster, and the severely impaired group didn't improve at all. Overall, rolfing decreased the subjects' passive range of motion (how far someone else can move your limbs, as opposed to how far *you* can) as often as it increased it. [Perry]

Trager bodywork

The *Trager* method of bodywork combines light, tension-releasing massage with a series of gentle, painless, passive movements that help patients expand their freedom of movement. In an uncontrolled study of twelve subjects with chronic lung disease, several measures of lung function improved after two weeks of Trager treatments. [Witt] It would be interesting to see whether a larger, controlled study would confirm these results.

Feldenkrais bodywork

To teach people to move their bodies more efficiently and comfortably, *Feldenkrais* bodywork uses highly structured movement sequences, with particular emphasis on head position. In a study of 30 normal subjects, those who performed a Feldenkrais sequence gained more flexibility in their necks than those who chose their own seated activity (reading, studying, etc.). But this result would be more convincing if the control group had performed some other kind of exercise, rather than an activity done while sitting. [Ruth]

Therapeutic touch

Therapeutic touch has been called a "healing meditation" in which energy is transferred from one person to another in order to potentiate the healing process. It's the secular version of the religious *laying on of hands,* but both terms are misnomers, since actual physical contact need not occur.

Therapeutic touch practitioners, in a meditative state, hold their hands on the skin or a short distance away from patients in order to sense—and smooth out—the patients' energy field. The technique is quite popular among nurses, perhaps because a nurse, Delores Krieger, popularized it. [Krieger]

Therapeutic touch does seem to have an effect on both humans and animals. Compared to casual touch or conversation, it was better at decreasing anxiety levels in hospitalized patients. [Heidt] Another study of 30 hospitalized children under two years of age found that, compared with casual touch, therapeutic touch reduced the time needed to calm children after stressful experiences. [Kramer]

A fascinating study looked at the effect of therapeutic touch on wounds that were the result of a biopsy on the upper arm. The 44 subjects stuck their injured arms through a hole in a door; half received a five-minute therapeutic touch session on the arm and half received no treatment. (The subjects, deliberately misled about the experiment, were told that they were being monitored by a machine.) The wounds of the group that was treated by therapeutic touch healed much more quickly than the untreated group's. [Wirth]

Several studies compared therapeutic touch to sham therapeutic touch, in which practitioners simulate the movements of therapeutic touch but don't concentrate on what they're doing (they may even do a distracting mental exercise, like counting backwards by sevens). One trial of 60 hospitalized patients found a greater decrease in anxiety among those who received real rather than sham therapeutic touch. [Quinn]

The effect of therapeutic touch on pain is less clear. In a study of 60 patients with tension headaches, real therapeutic touch reduced pain in 90% of the subjects, but sham treatment reduced it 80%. However, the patients who received the real treatment had a greater decrease in pain, and also used fewer pain medications in the four hours after the treatment. [Keller]

In another study of pain after surgery, a painkiller worked best, and therapeutic touch wasn't significantly better than sham therapeutic touch. There was, however, some indication that those who received therapeutic touch reduced their need for narcotic medications. [Meehan]

The inventor of therapeutic touch, Delores Krieger, studied under a Canadian healer named Oskar Estabany, and there are also a couple of interesting studies relating to his work. The wounds of mice healed much faster when they were treated by Estabany than when they were handled by nonhealers or simply warmed (to control for the heat of the healer's hands). [Grad, Benor] In another study, mice given a substance that causes goiters grew them much more slowly when they were treated by Estabany than when they weren't. [Benor]

Therapeutic touch and other types of energy healing appear to be a promising area for further research.

THE MIND/BODY CONNECTION

If the mind, which rules the body, ever forgets itself so far as to trample upon its slave, the slave is never generous enough to forgive the injury; but will rise and smite its oppressor. Longfellow, *Hyperion* (1839)

Give your brain as much attention as you do your hair and you'll be a thousand times better off.

Malcolm X, *Malcolm X on Afro-American History* (1967)

Mental health is intimately connected with physical health. A partial list of conditions affected by stress and other psychosomatic factors includes asthma, heart problems, gastrointestinal disorders, diseases of the musculoskeletal system, endocrine disorders, and obesity. [Cheren] (For more on the important topic of the mind's effect on the body, see the chapters on biofeedback, hypnosis and imagery, and relaxation and meditation.)

Relationships with other people and the feeling of belonging to a community are good for your health. A California study of 6928 adults found that men with the most social contacts were more than twice as like-ly—and women almost three times as likely—to be alive at a nine-year follow-up, compared to the most isolated men and women. [Berkman]

Another study of 2754 adults who were tracked for nine to twelve years found that men reporting a higher level of social relationships and activities were significantly more likely to be alive at the end of the tracking period. The more time subjects spent in solitary pastimes (watching TV, listening to the radio or reading), the higher their mortality rate. [House]

The effect of work

Just as you suspected, Mondays are bad for your health—more heart attacks occur on that day than any other day of the week. [Thompson] Saturday is the second most dangerous day (although to a much lesser extent). [Massing] Why would that be? It's thought that adjusting to anything new, even leisure, is stressful, so both starting the work week and starting the weekend are a strain on the heart. Or maybe the cause is Friday night carousing, if it includes heavy intake of alcohol and fatty foods.

What job you're showing up to also makes a difference. In addition to the level of job stress, the degree of autonomy and control you have at work is key. People in the highest-stress jobs with the least amount of control (for example, cooks, waiters, cashiers, people who work on assembly lines, nurse's aides, postal workers and office computer operators) had 3.8 to 4.8 times as many heart attacks as those in the lowest-stress, highest-control jobs (for example, architects, barbers, civil engineers, dentists, foresters, foremen, natural scientists, programmers, sales reps, social workers and therapists). The researchers who did this study point out that the risks of certain jobs are equivalent to the risks of smoking or having a high cholesterol level! [Karasek]

The effect of attitude

Chronic hostility, depression and repression have a negative effect on physical health. A study of 1877 employed men between the ages of 40 and 55 found that high levels of hostility correlated with higher rates of death from cardiovascular disease—and with higher rates of death from any cause. [Shekelle] Enthusiasm, on the other hand, correlates with the ability to recover from illness—enthusiastic people tend to have the most resilient, "self-healing" personalities. [Friedman]

It helps to laugh a lot too. Laughter raises endorphins (opiate-like hormones found mostly in the brain) and lowers cortisol (a stress-induced hormone). [FPN] One small study compared levels of various hormones in the blood of five healthy male controls with those of five healthy men who were shown a humorous video. The video group had decreased cortisol, epinephrine and other stress hormones, but in this study, there was no difference in endorphins. [Berk]

A researcher at the University of California points out that children laugh 400 times a day, while adults only laugh about 15 times a day. Maybe this explains why grown-ups have a higher mortality rate than children. [FPN]

The effect of expectations

In cultures that believe in spells and sorcery, numerous cases have been reported of someone dying within hours or days after being cursed or bewitched. [Cannon] Mortality studies have shown that death rates rise after events or holidays important to the people studied, perhaps indicating that individuals can will themselves to hold onto life for at least limited amounts of time. [Marriott, Phillips 1]

One study found that Chinese Americans who contract diseases considered unlucky for people born in their birth years (according to Chinese five-element theory) died earlier than European Americans born in the same years who contracted the same diseases. The major flaw of this study is that no effort was made to determine whether the Chinese Americans involved actually believed in, or knew about this particular application of, five-element theory. [Phillips 2]

While many proponents of behavioral therapies such as biofeedback, relaxation, hypnosis and meditation claim a beneficial effect on high blood pressure, a meta-analysis of controlled trials found that, while these therapies were superior to no treatment, they weren't superior to sham interventions. This excellent analysis points up the trap of claiming efficacy for therapies because they work better than nothing. Interventions must be compared with placebo treatments, because the expectations of patients improve any treatment. [Eisenberg]

The effect of music

Music can affect blood pressure and stress levels. Several studies show that music can help relieve pain. [Kerkvliet] One done in 1929 found that changes in blood pressure depended on volume, pitch, melody, rhythm and type of music, but that the strongest determining factor was comprehension of and interest in the music. [Vincent]

However, a study in a coronary care unit found that both silence and *white noise* ("synthetic silence" created by sound on all wave lengths, similar to ocean waves) were as effective in lowering physiological stress responses as was music selected by the patients. The authors conclude that the actual therapeutic intervention was simply 30 minutes of uninterrupted rest. [Zimmerman]

A study of surgeons who regularly listen to music in the operating room showed a different result. It found that physiological stress responses were decreased and a stressful task was performed better when the surgeons selected the music themselves than when they listened to music selected by someone else, or to no music at all. [Allen]

(A friend of the editor's emerged from surgery with Beach Boys music running through her head. After a couple of days of not being able to get rid of it, she called her doctor, who broke into laughter and told her that that's what they'd been playing in the operating room. Even though she'd been under general anesthesia, the music had penetrated her subconscious and persisted after she woke up.)

Effects on the cardiovascular system
For patients who've had a heart attack, living alone increases the risk of having another. In 1234 patients followed for one to four years, those living alone at the time of their heart attack were 50% more likely to have another heart attack, compared to those living with one or more other people. At six months, the risk

was even higher—16% for those living alone vs. 9% for those living with other people. [Case]

Psychological stress can cause adverse changes in heart rhythms in dogs, pigs and humans. [Lown] Public speaking caused an irregular heart rhythm in 6 out of 23 healthy individuals and 5 out of 7 people with coronary artery disease. [Taggart 1] Driving in traffic also affects the heartbeat. [Taggart 2]

In another study, patients with cardiovascular disease were subjected to mental stress, induced by tasks such as counting backwards by sevens, or giving a five-minute speech about their faults. They developed changes in heart function that indicated decreased oxygen flow to the heart muscle. [Rozanski]

Effects on immunity

Separation, divorce, bereavement, an unhappy marriage and taking care of someone who's ill have all been shown to affect not only emotional health but also immunity. Stress is a factor in both the development and recurrence of herpes and Epstein-Barr viral infections. [Kiecolt-Glaser 1] In a study of 75 medical students, there was a significant decrease in natural killer cells, an important part of the immune system, in blood drawn on the first day of exams, compared to blood drawn a month earlier. [Kiecolt-Glaser 2]

Healthy college students participated in a study of imagery, music and immune function. One group was given a lecture on the immune system and then listened to a tape of instructions and music meant to enhance imagery. The second group only listened to music, and the third group received no intervention. Both the imagery group and the music-only group were able to significantly increase their secretory IgA (a component of the immune system), compared with students who did neither. [Rider]

In another study, thirteen people who cared for loved ones with Alzheimer's disease were compared to thirteen age- and income-matched controls. In all subjects, a small chunk was taken out of the forearm with a punch biopsy instrument. Healing was assessed by photographs and by whether hydrogen peroxide foamed on contact with the wound. The caregivers' wounds took an average of 49 days to heal, compared to 39 days for the controls. [Kiecolt-Glaser 3]

A related study found that Alzheimer's caregivers had a decreased response to flu vaccine up to two years after their patients had died, showing that adverse effects on the immune system may persist long after the stress is removed. [Flach]

In thirteen patients with Stage 1 breast cancer (that hasn't reached the lymph nodes), a combination of relaxation, guided imagery and biofeedback had a positive effect on the immune system, including an increase in natural killer cells and a type of white blood cell called lymphocytes. [Gruber]

Effects on cancer survival

Psychotherapy, group therapy, relaxation and imagery appeared to extend median survival time in 225 cancer patients, compared to standard survival times. Although this trial didn't utilize a control group (comparing to standard survival times is very problematic and doesn't count as a control), it's one of the first trials of psychological intervention with cancer patients and deserves to be mentioned. [Simonton]

In patients with metastatic breast cancer, weekly support groups and self-hypnosis for pain doubled length of survival. The 50 patients in the support group survived about 37 months while the 36 in the control group survived an average of 19 months. [Spiegel 2]

Effects on pain

Fifty-four women with metastatic breast cancer were given weekly group therapy, either with or without self-hypnosis training. Both treatment groups had less suffering and less intensity of pain, but there was no difference in frequency or duration of pain. The group that did the self-hypnosis training was better able to control the intensity of pain. [Spiegel 1]

In patients who'd previously been trained in biofeedback, warming imagery directed at the painful trigger points of fibromyalgia increased skin temperature and muscle relaxation and also decreased sensitivity to pressure. [Albright]

Effects on irritable bowel syndrome

Psychological treatment can help people with irritable bowel syndrome (IBS). A study of 102 patients whose symptoms hadn't improved after six months of standard medical treatment divided them into two groups. Both continued to receive standard medical treatment, but one group also received psychotherapy and relaxation exercises. After three months, the psychological-ly treated group had less abdominal pain and diar-rhea—although constipation didn't improve. [Guthrie]

In a randomized trial of 35 patients with IBS, a stress-management program that included breathing exercis-es was more effective than an antispasmodic drug. [Shaw] In an uncontrolled study, 27 patients with IBS were trained in progressive muscle relaxation, biofeedback and cognitive therapy, and were educated about their disease. At a four-year follow-up, 89% of the patients showed more than a 50% improvement. [Schwartz]

RELAXATION AND MEDITATION

Relaxation and meditation are two related therapies that have been quite successful in dealing with a number of medical conditions. Some relaxation techniques use pleasant imagery, but many of the studies described here use progressive relaxation training *(PRT)*.

In PRT, subjects divide their muscles into seven groups and then learn to tense and relax each group in turn. Later they learn to relax muscles in four groups and, finally, to release tension in all of their muscles at once.

Meditation is a process in which one tries to achieve awareness without thought. Formal sitting meditation is the best-known approach, but it's also possible to meditate while walking, cooking or watching the night sky.

Practitioners of *mindfulness* meditation learn to pay nonjudgmental, moment-to-moment attention to the changing objects of perception and cognition. [Miller] In contrast, practitioners of Transcendental Meditation focus on a single object, or on a word or short phrase called a *mantra*. (For more on TM, see the end of the chapter.)

Can meditation have negative effects? In a study of long-term meditators who were interviewed before and after either a two-week or a three-month silent meditation retreat, 17 out of 27 reported at least one adverse effect (negativity, disorientation, worsened interpersonal relationships or increased alienation from society). Two experienced such discomfort that they stopped meditating (one had taken the three-month retreat, the other the two-week).

However, many more of the subjects (89% before the retreat, 81% one month after and 92% six months after) reported that meditation reduced their stress and increased their happiness, self-confidence and effectiveness. [Shapiro] Nevertheless, in patients with a predisposition to mental illness, meditation may worsen symptoms. [Walsh, Lazarus]

Seizures

Numerous studies confirm that relaxation techniques are effective ways to reduce the frequency of seizures. The first controlled trial of PRT and seizures treated eight patients with poorly controlled epilepsy. Four learned PRT; the other four first received a sham treatment, then PRT. The sham treatment had no effect, but PRT resulted in a 30% reduction in the median frequency of seizures in both groups. [Rousseau]

In a similar study of 24 epilepsy patients, PRT reduced seizure frequency by 29%. In a control group that practiced quiet sitting, seizure frequency dropped only 3%. [Puskarich]

In an uncontrolled study of twelve patients, PRT decreased seizure frequency by 21% after two months and 54% after six months. (Most progressive relaxation techniques are taught in ten training sessions, but this study only used three.) [Whitman]

In another study, eighteen epileptic adults were divided into three groups: one learned to relax their muscles, identify high-risk situations and apply learned relaxation techniques to them; the second received supportive therapy; and the third merely recorded how often they had seizures. Initially, only the first group showed a significant decrease in the frequency of seizures. In the second part of the study, however, both the control groups were also taught relaxation techniques—at which point their seizure frequency decreased significantly. [Dahl 2]

In another study by the same investigator, eighteen children with severe epilepsy were assigned to one of three groups: behavioral and relaxation training, "no treatment" or "attention only." In ten-week and one-year follow-up studies, only the relaxation group showed a reduction in the "seizure index" (which evaluates both the number and duration of seizures). [Dahl 1]

Meditation's ability to reduce stress and anxiety may also help with seizures. In a small study, eleven epileptics whose seizures were inadequately controlled by drugs practiced meditation for twenty minutes a day for a year. They had fewer and shorter seizures and showed improvements in their EEGs (brain wave measurements), while controls showed no changes. [Deepak]

Anxiety

In an uncontrolled study, 22 patients with generalized anxiety or panic disorder participated in an eight-week intensive stress-reduction program that emphasized meditation. Both patients and therapists submitted assessments weekly before and during the program, then monthly during the follow-up period.

Twenty patients scored significantly lower in anxiety and depression immediately after treatment. [Kabat-Zinn 2] In a three-year follow-up, with most of the patients still meditating, 18 of the 20 who sent in assessments showed continued improvement in their anxiety and depression scores, and had fewer and less severe panic attacks. [Miller]

Mood

One hundred fifty-four breast cancer patients receiving radiation therapy were assigned at random to one of three treatments: progressive muscle relaxation and deep breathing, relaxation and deep breathing with pleasant imagery, or a control group whose members were simply encouraged to talk about themselves. Before the study, all of the subjects shared similar scores in self-rated measures of mood, depression and anxiety. After six weeks, the first two groups had significantly better mood scores (subjects in the relaxation and imagery group did best), while mood scores were worst in the control group. (There were no differences in depression and anxiety, however.) [Bridge]

Another study randomly assigned 24 patients scheduled to have their gallbladders removed to one of two groups. The first observed 20 minutes of quiet time daily for five days (starting the day before surgery); the second watched a 20-minute videotape on relaxation and guided imagery for the same period. Subjects in the second group showed less anxiety following surgery than the controls. [Holden-Lund]

Pain

For patients with chronic low-back pain, relaxation training was found to be better at reducing pain and muscle tension than placebos or EMG biofeedback (described in the biofeedback chapter). [Stuckey] In an uncontrolled study of 225 patients with chronic pain who were taught mindfulness meditation, 60% reported moderate or great improvement after four years. [Kabat-Zinn 1]

In another study, 50 patients received a single hour of relaxation instruction the evening before spinal surgery. Compared to 50 other patients scheduled for the same operation (who were matched for gender, etc.), the relaxation group had shorter hospital stays and used less pain medication, and complained less to nurses. [Lawlis]

In a controlled trial of 42 patients hospitalized for various kinds of elective surgery, the half that learned the Jacobson relaxation technique—in which subjects attempt to drop their jaws, relax their tongues, make their breathing rhythmical and regular and ignore thoughts and words—used fewer painkillers, reported less pain and had more relaxed breathing patterns after surgery. [Flaherty]

In a controlled study of 20 elderly adults who'd undergone surgery for a fractured hip, the half who learned the Jacobson technique reported less pain and used fewer painkillers when they were turned in their beds from their back to their sides (within 24 hours after surgery). [Ceccio]

Effects on trauma

In one study of severe orthopedic trauma—gunshot wounds, crushed ankles, etc.—64 patients were divided into four groups. The groups that received audio-taped relaxation training or relaxation plus biofeedback had less discomfort and anxiety, and lower systolic blood pressure, than the attention-only or control groups. [Achterberg]

Immunity

In a study of 45 elderly people in independent living facilities, one group received relaxation training three times a week, one group received social contact three times a week, and the third group received no contact. After a month, the relaxation group showed a significant increase in natural killer cell activity; antibody levels of herpes virus also dropped, and the subjects reported feeling more relaxed. There were no significant changes in the groups that got social contact or no contact. [Kiecolt-Glaser]

TM

Maharishi Mahesh Yogi popularized Transcendental Meditation, or TM, in the United States in the 1970s. (He later developed a form of ayurvedic medicine; for more on that, see the chapter on ayurveda.) Because the Maharishi and his followers comprise a well-funded movement that supports its own research, there's more literature on TM than on other forms of meditation that may be equally—or more—beneficial. My own impression is that most TM studies are poorly done but well-written.

Maharishi followers often quote a study that claims that TM practitioners used fewer medical services than other people covered by the same insurance carrier. The study is flawed, however, because it ignored age differences between the two groups (obviously, the older you are, the more likely you are to visit a doctor), as well as other confounding factors like diet, prior medical illnesses, and use of alcohol and tobacco. [Orme-Johnson]

Another study claimed that TM practitioners have lower blood pressure than the norms for the general population. However, the TM study participants rested for five to ten minutes before having their blood pressure taken. This isn't normally done, and lowers blood pressure significantly.

Also, only systolic blood pressure—the top number on a reading—was measured. Diastolic pressure—the bottom number—is more important in predicting the risk of cardiovascular disease, and it also fluctuates much less.

For such a study to be meaningful, both diastolic and systolic blood pressure would have to be taken, the two groups would have to be matched in terms of age, sex and pre-existing high blood pressure, and the controls would have to have the same rest period before measurement as the TM group. [Wallace]

A meta-analysis of studies on relaxation techniques found that PRT, EMG biofeedback and various forms of meditation were all effective in treating *trait anxiety* (the general tendency to be anxious), but that TM was the most effective. [Eppley] However, this conclusion hasn't been borne out in other trials.

In a well-performed study, 49 anxious college students were taught either to do TM or to sit quietly with their eyes closed. (The researchers went to great lengths to blind this study. They dreamt up a name for the placebo activity of sitting quietly—*PSI*, for *periodic somatic inactivity*—and even had PSI logos, and phony PSI studies, made up to show to the subjects. The even convinced the PSI *instructor* that PSI was a real thing.) After six months, both the TM and the "PSI" group had improved equally. [Smith]

In a related study, 27 students learned a TM-like meditation technique (from someone who wasn't an official TM teacher), while 27 others were instructed to fantasize about a positive situation, mentally list the positive attributes of something, or tell themselves a positive story. Although this amount of mental activity is antithetical to meditation, here again, both groups improved. [Smith]

SPIRITUAL HEALING
AND ENERGY WORK

As the chapter on the mind/body connection makes clear, one's thoughts, feelings, emotions and expectations can have profound effects on one's health. For this reason alone, prayers for health may help the person praying. The social support that comes from worshipping with others may also be beneficial.

Given that, it's somewhat surprising that scientific evidence for the power of prayer is virtually nonexistent. Sir Frances Galton, the 19th-century English scientist, quoted studies to the effect that sovereigns, who are prayed for regularly, are the shortest-lived people in the affluent classes, and that the clergy, who presumably pray more often than others, don't live significantly longer than doctors or lawyers. [Galton]

A more recent review of 27 studies found that, in 22 of them, frequency of attendance at religious services was associated with better health. [Levin] Unfortunately, most of these studies were uncontrolled and had other methodological problems. If the religious people shared other traits as well—if, say, they exercised as much as they worshipped, or sought solace in religion rather than in cigarettes or alcohol—religion might have nothing to do with their improved health. Still, this area merits further study.

There have been some decent studies on *therapeutic touch,* the secular version of the laying-on of hands; they're described in the massage and bodywork chap-

175

ter. But research on *distant healing*—having strangers send energy towards you, or pray or meditate for you—is, to be generous, unconvincing. The same is true of *directed healing*—"intention" affecting everything from enzymes to plants. In both these areas, the studies tend to demonstrate the saying that if you torture your data enough, it will tell you anything.

Directed healing

A survey of 131 controlled trials on various healers' effects on enzymes, cells, bacteria, fungi and plants claims that 43% of these trials were positive. Even taken at face value, this isn't too impressive, since it means that 57%—more than half of the studies—were negative. But even that's exaggerated, since many more of the trials were negative than the author of the survey was willing to admit. For example, although he described one study as having insufficient data, and although all attempted reruns of it were negative, he counted it as questionably positive.

Of five experiments done with another healer, only one was positive, but that was enough to get the whole five-experiment trial labeled positive. In a study of the effect of a third healer on an enzyme in red blood cells, enzyme activity increased in nine trials, decreased in seven and was unchanged in two, but these results—inconclusive at best—were also counted as positive. [Benor 2]

A book by the same author suffers from the same problems. When experiments don't come out positively, it's attributed to stress on the part of the healer, and the experiments are often repeated over and over until the desired result is obtained. The research approach seems to be: put a chimp at a typewriter long enough and he'll produce a novel—or, to put it another way, even a stopped clock is right twice a day. [Benor 1]

Distant healing

No research to date supports the claim that distant healing—also called *intercessory prayer*—works. A study often cited as proof that prayer had an effect on the health of 393 patients in a coronary care unit is badly flawed in a couple of ways.

One problem was there were significant differences between the two groups other than that one was prayed for and the other wasn't. People end up in a coronary care unit for many reasons, from a severe heart attack to gastrointestinal bleeding (which, while easily treated, can eventually cause irregularities in heart rhythms). In this study, more people in the control group came in with relatively serious conditions like acute heart attack or unstable angina, and more people in the treated group came in with relatively minor conditions like fainting, chest pain of unknown cause or gastrointestinal bleeding (10% of the prayed-for group had this last condition vs. only 3% of the controls).

Another problem with this study was that measurement of results was idiosyncratic to the point of absurdity. For example, no distinction was made between death and having to have cardiac surgery—both were classed simply as "bad" outcomes. Of the 26 new problems, diagnoses and other events that were looked at, only 6 showed any difference between prayed-for patients and controls. On measures that couldn't be played with—death, for example, or days in the hospital, or in the cardiac care unit, after entering the study—prayer made no difference. To call this study positive is to torture data until it screams. [Byrd]

Another trial looked at the effect of prayer in sixteen pairs of patients with a variety of psychological and rheumatic diseases. (I'm not sure why they put these two categories together.) No significant effect was found, although the researchers attempted to put a positive spin on the results anyway—by blaming the small sample size and saying that their results almost reached significance. [Joyce]

In one of the least convincing prayer studies, eight out of eighteen leukemic children were prayed for and a positive effect on survival was claimed. However, the children weren't matched in terms of their age, how far along their disease was, what medical treatment they'd received, or even what type of leukemia they had. [Collipp]

A prospective, randomized trial divided 115 subjects with high blood pressure into three groups. One received laying-on of hands, another received distant healing and the third got no treatment. After fifteen weeks, both systolic and diastolic blood pressure dropped in all three groups; no treatment was found to be consistently superior to another. [Beutler]

Better research needs to be done to examine whether there's any scientific validity to the claim that prayer can influence health. My own prediction is that distant healing doesn't work unless the subject knows about it and believes in it—in other words, that it's basically placebo effect.

Spiritism

Spiritism—often known by its Spanish name, *espiritismo*—is a healing system that originated in the 19th-century French writings of Leon H. Rivail, who wrote under the pseudonym Allan Kardec. Spiritism is now a popular form of healing in Cuba, and it's estimated that 60% of the people in Puerto Rico have visited a spiritist center at least once.

In one Puerto Rican study, patients who saw spiritists were more satisfied with the results than those who received mental health services. (The study didn't measure efficacy of treatment, just patients' satisfaction.) [Koss]

MISCELLANEOUS THERAPIES

This chapter gathers up several loose ends not covered elsewhere in the book, but there are many other alternative therapies on which scientific research simply hasn't been done. We need trials on bee pollen for allergies, bee stings for arthritis or multiple sclerosis, saw palmetto for enlarged prostates, acupuncture for infertility, ozone therapy for AIDS...the list goes on.

Whether or not one believes in these alternatives, their safety and efficacy should be studied simply as a public health issue, since they're being used by thousands of patients. If a new therapy is more effective than a conventional one, or is equally effective but causes fewer side effects, it should be the treatment of choice. On the other hand, if a therapy is ineffective or dangerous, consumers should be informed of that as well.

Alternative cancer therapies

One of the areas in which there's an appalling dearth of clinical trials is alternative cancer treatments. When I coordinated field investigations at the Office of Alternative Medicine at the National Institutes of Health, I saw a number of intriguing approaches to cancer, including herbal and metabolic therapies, that clearly should be studied in clinical trials.

Two studies that have been done both came out negative for the alternative treatments looked at. One compared 78 cancer patients who received Livingston-Wheeler therapy (immune-enhancing vaccines, a vegetarian diet, coffee enemas and injections of an antitu-berculosis vaccine called bacille Calmette-Guerin) with a control group that only received conventional care (some of the Livingston-Wheeler patients were also receiving conventional therapy). There was no difference in survival between the two groups, and quality-of-life measures were better among the conventionally treated patients. [Cassileth]

A controlled, double-blind study compared 60 patients who took ten grams of vitamin C daily with 63 patients who took a placebo. There was no difference between the two groups in symptoms, weight or survival. But note that these were terminal patients—their average survival time was only seven weeks. A common criticism of this study is that it was undertaken too late to do these patients any good. [Creagan]

Applied kinesiology

In applied kinesiology—also called *muscle testing*—a patient's baseline muscle strength is tested, usually by having him hold his arm out straight and resist the practitioner's attempt to push it down. Then a substance is placed in the patient's other hand (typically in a sealed glass vial), or placed on his skin or under his tongue, and the practitioner tries to push his arm down again. If the patient's resistance is weaker, this is said to mean that the substance being tested isn't good for him

Applied kinesiology is not only used for diagnosis but also to test remedies. If a given remedy increases muscle strength, it's appropriate; if it decreases muscle strength, it isn't.

In a study unusual for the fact that the applied kinesiology practitioners were blinded but the patients weren't, 73 men were divided into two groups. One group had sugar cubes in their mouths; the other didn't. (Refined sugar is said to weaken the muscles.) The practitioners said that 48% of the men with sugar in their mouths were weakened vs. only 13% of the controls.

However, a *mechanical* test of muscle strength showed no difference between the two groups. This may mean that practitioners are more sensitive to varying muscle strength than machines, or that they somehow figured out who had sugar in their mouths from subconsciously noted clues and imagined changes in muscle strength that weren't really there. [Rybeck]

Another controlled trial used muscle testing as a diagnostic screen for supplemental nutrition therapy. Fifty patients whose latissimus dorsi muscles applied kinesiologists determined to be weak had either an active substance or a placebo placed on their abdomen or under their tongue; then their muscle strength was tested again. Subjects who'd been given the active treatment were no stronger than those who'd been given the inactive treatments. [Triano]

Aromatherapy

Although it may seem obvious that pleasant or unpleasant smells can affect our moods—the aroma of baking bread or apple pie taking you back to your grandmother's kitchen, or a perfumed envelope reminding you of a lover—the effect can be highly individualized. The smell of a madeleine brought a rush of memories to Proust, but that rather bland, cookie-sized, seashell-shaped sponge cake probably wouldn't inspire most of us in the same way.

Odors most people find pleasant may also have unpleasant connotations for others. In my anatomy class in medical school, the cadavers we dissected had been soaked in formaldehyde to which mint had been added. Later I worked in a hospital where peppermint oil was used to cover up the smell of vomit or feces on inadequately cleaned floors. So for me, the smell of mint brings back disgusting memories.

A number of studies have looked at whether exposure to certain odors affects human performance, but results have been mixed: studies of pleasant odors have shown no effect, [Knasko 2, Kirk-Smith, Baron] positive effects [Warm] or negative effects. [Ludvigson] One particularly interesting study compared 90 subjects exposed to the scent of lemon or ylang-ylang (from a tropical Asian tree) with those exposed to unpleasant smells or to no smell. Although tests and questionnaires measuring task performance, mood and perceived health found no actual difference among the three groups, those exposed to the unpleasant smells thought they were adversely affected by all of these factors. [Knasko 2]

Another study by the same researcher tested subjects on creativity, mood and perceived health, and then gave them the same tests a week later. The room in which the subjects were tested was unscented during one session and scented with lemon, lavender or DMS (dimethyl sulfide, which has an unpleasant odor) during the other.

Those in the lemon group reported fewer health complaints on scented vs. unscented days (perhaps because we associate lemon with cleanliness). Those in the lavender group tended to be in a better mood than those in the DMS group. Those exposed to DMS in the first session were in a much worse mood during the second session, even though the room was unscented—perhaps because the memory of being in an unpleasant-smelling room was depressing. [Knasko 1]

Inhaling vapor from black pepper extract can reduce smoking withdrawal symptoms. Forty-eight cigarette smokers were deprived of cigarettes overnight, then divided into three groups and given devices to puff on for three hours (no smoking was allowed). To the first group, the device delivered the smell of black pepper; to the second group, the smell of mint; and to the third group, just unscented air.

The subjects then filled out a questionnaire rating the experience. (In addition, they'd been filling out questionnaires every hour that rated their mood and how much they craved cigarettes.) Both black pepper and mint improved the subjects' mood and got higher satisfaction ratings than plain air, but craving for cigarettes was significantly reduced only in the black pepper group (as were symptoms of anxiety). [Rose]

Given all this evidence for the effect of various smells, it's not surprising that there's a type of alternative medical treatment based on them. Called *aromatherapy,* it holds that scents, even unfamiliar ones, can trigger emotions, and that the proper use of scents can have health benefits.

Aromatherapists use essential oils distilled from plants—never animal, mineral or synthetic ingredients. These essential oils are either inhaled from a handkerchief, put in bath water, mixed into skin products or massage oil, or diffused into the air by means of a ceramic ring placed around a light bulb (or with more complicated devices).

Many aromatherapists claim that any use of an essential oil falls under aromatherapy, but when an essential oil is taken internally, or used at high concentrations on the skin, herbalists clearly have an equal claim to the bailiwick. (For information on other uses of essential oils, see the section on them below.)

Probably the most common use of aromatherapy is during a massage. Massage is very relaxing by itself, of course, and most studies that have compared massage with and without aromatherapy haven't found large differences between the two groups. But at least one good study has shown some additional effect from aromatherapy.

Fifty-one cancer patients in a hospice were divided into two groups. Anxiety decreased somewhat in the group that received three massages with plain almond oil, but the group that received three aromatherapy massages (with 1% of an essential oil called roman chamomile added to the massage oil) had even less anxiety, fewer physical symptoms and better quality of life. [Wilkinson]

In another study of patients who'd undergone heart surgery, a group who received foot massage with plain oil reported more anxiety and less relaxation at a five-day follow-up than a group who received the same foot massage with neroli (orange) oil added to the massage oil. [Stevenson]

Aromatherapy also has uses beyond massage. For example, jasmine can suppress lactation. This is important, because women who choose not to nurse, or who stop nursing, can be very uncomfortable for weeks.

The drug commonly used to suppress lactation is bromocriptine, which can cause strokes and seizures. What's more, it doesn't always have a permanent effect; some women resume lactating when they're taken off it.

In Kerala (at the southern tip of India), women traditionally tape jasmine flowers *(Jasminum sambac)* to their breasts to suppress lactation. In a study of 60 women in southern India, this technique worked as well as bromocriptine. [Shrivastav]

There's also a fascinating animal study of jasmine. Twelve lactating mice were divided into a control group, a group exposed to the smell of jasmine flowers and a group whose cages were lined with jasmine flowers, so that their mammary glands would come in contact with the flowers as they crawled around. Baby mice were weighed before and after suckling, and the mother mice were weighed as well, in order to determine how much milk was being produced.

The mice whose cages were lined with jasmine flowers produced only an eighth as much milk as the controls, and mice exposed to the odor of jasmine produced about half as much as controls. Microscopic examination of the mammary glands showed changes in mice who smelled the jasmine odor and even more marked changes in the mice who crawled around on the jasmine flowers. [Abraham]

Not all aromatherapy is effective. A blinded randomized trial of 635 women tested the effect of putting lavender in bath water on soreness or pain in the perineum after giving birth. Neither pure nor synthetic lavender oil helped the discomfort better than a placebo that was aromatic but smelled nothing like lavender. [Dale]

A recent book contains a thorough discussion of the practice of massage and aromatherapy, as well as a critique of research on the subject. Readers who want more depth on this subject are referred to it. [Vickers]

Chelation

The drug EDTA (ethylenediamine tetraacetic acid) is used to treat lead poisoning because it grabs onto lead (as well as other minerals), thus allowing the body to excrete them. This process is called *chelation*.

Since 1955, chelation with EDTA has also been used as an alternative treatment for cardiovascular disease and peripheral vascular disease (blockage or narrowing of blood vessels in the legs), although not by conventional doctors. The theory is that the EDTA removes calcium from atherosclerotic lesions in the arteries.

There have been many studies on this approach, but a comprehensive review found that few of them were controlled, and fewer yet double-blind. Although some of the trials showed a temporary improvement in angina, neither long-term improvement of exercise tolerance nor reductions in death rates have been convincingly demonstrated. [Grier]

Two double-blind, placebo-controlled trials have been done of chelation therapy for intermittent claudication (pain on walking that's caused by peripheral vascular disease)—one with 32 patients [van Rij] and another with 153. [Guldager] In both studies, chelation failed to increase the distance patients could walk without pain.

DHEA

DHEA (dehydroepiandrosterone), a steroid hormone produced by the adrenal glands, is currently being touted as an anti-aging, anticancer miracle supplement. While DHEA is the most common steroid hormone in the blood, its role has not been well-defined. [Ebeling]

(DHEA also comes in a bound, storage form: DHEA-sulfate, or *DHEA-S*. The ratio of DHEA to DHEA-S is constant throughout one's life, so you can more or less ignore which one is being talked about in the studies cited below.)

Levels of DHEA-S in the blood peak at 20–24 years of age; in each subsequent decade, they fall to 80% of the previous decade's level. By age 85–90, the DHEA-S level averages about 10% of the 20-year-old level. [Regelson]

A retrospective study of 49 men who'd had early heart attacks (before the age of 56) found that their levels of DHEA-S were much lower than 49 age-matched controls. [Mitchell] According to one study, high levels of DHEA-S seem to correlate with less cardiovascular disease in men, [Barrett-Connor 2] but in women, high levels seem to correlate with *increased* risk. [Barrett-Connor 1]

A small, uncontrolled study of ten patients with lupus (also called systemic lupus erythematosus, or SLE—an autoimmune disease that can cause arthritis, fatigue, fever, rash, skin lesions and kidney problems) found that three to six months of DHEA treatment improved symptoms of the disease, in the opinion of both the patients themselves and their physicians. [van Vollenhoven]

In patients with HIV disease, decreased DHEA levels are seen in those with more advanced illness. [Wisniewski] Premenopausal breast cancer patients seem to have lower levels of DHEA-S than their peers, [Zumoff] but postmenopausal breast cancer patients have *higher* levels. [Gordon] DHEA may also cause acne and increased body hair in women. [van Vollenhoven]

There's enough intriguing evidence about DHEA that more studies should be done on it. But, in my view, there isn't a sufficient basis for recommending administration of this powerful hormone for preventive purposes or as drug therapy. DHEA shouldn't be regarded as a dietary supplement, but rather as a potent drug that may increase rates of cancer and heart disease in women. However, there are no studies showing long-term harmful effects in men.

Electromagnetic fields

The use of TENS *(transcutaneous electrical nerve stimulation)* machines to treat pain is an example of an alternative therapy that has crossed over into conventional medicine. There are other uses of electro-magnetic fields that should be explored as well.

A review of studies on various kinds of connective tissue repair found that electric and magnetic fields helped heal fractures, strengthen bones weakened by osteoporosis, repair cartilage and soft fibrous tissues, and incorporate bone grafts. [Aaron] A review of studies on nonhealing wounds found positive results for low-intensity direct current, low-frequency pulsed cur-rents, high voltage pulsed currents, pulsed electromagnetic fields, and stimulation of acupunc-ture points by TENS. Nonhealing wounds are a major problem for diabetics and other people with poor cir-culation, so this promising therapy should be explored further. [Vodovnik]

Pressure ulcers (also known as *pressure sores* or *bedsores)* are a serious problem in immobile patients. They start as redness on the heels or another part of the body; then the skin may break down, followed in some cases by a breakdown of the underlying tissues. Pressure sores are notoriously hard to heal, and increase the risk of infection until they're healed.

In one randomized, double-blind study of 30 male patients with spinal cord injuries at a Veteran's Administration hospital in New York, pulsed electro-magnetic energy treatment was administered to half the group for thirty minutes twice daily for twelve weeks (or until the pressure ulcer was healed); a dummy machine was used on the other half of the group. After a week, 84% of the pressure sores in the treated group had healed vs. 40% in the untreated group. [Salzberg]

In a randomized, double-blind study of 40 patients who'd had part of their shins removed to treat degeneration of the knee joint, half the group was treated with electromagnetic field stimulation; machines used on the control group had been deactivated. After two months, four orthopedic surgeons looked at X-rays and rated bone healing, placing people in four categories. Of the treated patients, 72% were rated as being in the most healed or next most healed category, vs. 26% of those in the control group. [Mammi]

In another randomized, double-blind trial of 47 patients who underwent bone grafts after having surgery for bone cancer, pulsed electromagnetic fields didn't shorten overall healing time, affect patient survival or prevent tumor recurrence. However, patients in the treated group who didn't undergo chemotherapy after surgery shortened their healing time from about 41 weeks to 29 weeks. [Capanna]

Electrical stimulation may also help ankle sprains. In a randomized, double-blind study of 50 active-duty troops with Grade I or II (mild to moderate) sprained ankles, one treatment with pulsed electromagnetic energy resulted in a statistically significant decrease in swelling. [Pennington]

Electromagnetic energy may even help nerves regenerate after injury, although this use isn't as well studied as the repair of wounds and of bones. [Sisken] Diabetes, heart attack, stroke, nerve damage and even cancer are all conditions that may be treated with electrical stimulation sometime in the future. [Bassett 1]

Essential oils

Aside from their use in aromatherapy (discussed above), essential oils from plants are sometimes taken internally, or are used in high concentrations on the skin. The dental profession seems to be far more comfortable with this than the medical profession. Oil of clove is often used in dental offices, and perhaps the most popular use of essential oils in the United States is in mouthwashes, like Listerine, that contain essential oils of thyme, mint and eucalyptus.

In an uncontrolled trial, capsules of essential oil of lemongrass (a tropical grass from southern India and Sri Lanka) were ingested by patients with high cholesterol. There was a modest average effect—cholesterol levels went from 310 to 294—but the treatment only seemed to work in some subjects.

When patients were divided into "responders" and "nonresponders", however, the differences were more marked; responders' cholesterol levels dropped 25 points in one month, 33 points in two months and 38 points in three months. After the treatment was withdrawn, cholesterol levels slowly drifted back up to their original levels. [Elson]

Irritable bowel syndrome (IBS) has been treated by giving peppermint oil capsules orally, with mixed results. Two double-blind, crossover trials showed a beneficial effect, [Rees, Dew] but a placebo-controlled, noncrossover study found no effect. [Nash]

An oral preparation of mixed essential oils (including peppermint and pine) appeared to dissolve gallstones in several uncontrolled trials, both when used with [Ellis 2, Sommerville] and without [Bell, Ellis 1] a cholesterol-dissolving drug. Menthol (an essential oil of peppermint) may have been the key component in the above mixture, since a controlled, double-blind trial found that the dosage of UDCA (ursodeoxycholic acid, a drug that helps to dissolve cholesterol gallstones) can be lowered when supplemented with menthol, without lowering the rate of gallstone dissolution. [Leuschner]

One double-blind, randomized, controlled study looked at the effect on headaches of two essential oils that are found in many skin rubs and throat lozenges. Topical preparations containing peppermint—either alone or in combination with eucalyptus—relaxed the temple muscles and also improved concentration. [Gobel]

The tree *Melaleuca alternifolia,* which grows only in Australia, was discovered—for the European world—by Captain Cook. After observing aborigines brewing the leaves of this plant into a medicinal tea, he gave the plant its common name—the *tea tree.* (It's no relation to the varieties of camellia used to brew regular tea.) In World War I, tea tree oil was included in the first-aid kits of Australian soldiers, for use on burns, bites and infections.

Tea tree oil is widely used as an antibacterial and antifungal topical medication, and several studies indicate its effectiveness. One compared pure tea tree oil and the antifungal drug clotrimazole for the treatment of fungal infection of the toenails. After six months, the two treatments were found to be equally effective. [Buck]

Another study compared the effectiveness against acne of 5% benzoyl peroxide lotion and 5% tea tree oil. Both treatments reduced acne lesions; benzoyl peroxide was more effective, but tea tree oil had fewer side effects. Actually, it's remarkable that tea tree oil had *any* effect at this concentration, since a 5% solution of it is very weak. It's typically used at full strength on the skin. [Bassett 2]

Essential oils should only be taken orally under the supervision of a practitioner experienced in their use. Tea tree oil and eucalyptus oil have been associated with childhood poisonings, [Jacobs, Webb] and ingestion of pennyroyal oil has killed at least two adults. [Sullivan, Vallance] Essential oils are safe to use topically if diluted (and a few are safe full-strength).

Melatonin
Melatonin is an intriguing hormone that regulates circadian (daily wake-sleep) rhythms. It's produced mostly by the pineal gland and in the gut (where its production appears to be controlled by nutritional factors, especially the availability of tryptophan, an amino acid precursor of melatonin). [Huether]

When we sleep, melatonin levels rise. But this rise, is stunted by the presence of even a tiny amount of light, such as a street light shining in a window. Alcohol consumption also blunts melatonin surges, which may explain why alcohol causes sleep disturbances. [Ekman]

There's evidence that melatonin helps jet lag, sleep quality and workers' tolerance for working odd and/or varying shifts. Nightly melatonin surges may even be protective against cancer, so the light pollution urban dwellers live with may put us at higher risk of that disease.

A small, placebo-controlled study of police officers working night shifts found that five mgs of melatonin taken at the desired bedtime helped the officers sleep and increased their alertness during working hours. [Folkard] In a double-blind, placebo-controlled, crossover trial of twelve elderly people who complained of insomnia, two mgs of melatonin nightly for three weeks helped the quality of sleep, although it didn't increase the amount of time spent sleeping. [Garfinkel]

In a double-blind trial of 52 flight crew members, one group took a placebo, another took five mgs of melatonin from three days before arrival till five days after, and the third group took a placebo for three days, then melatonin for five days. The group that took the placebo, then melatonin, reported less jet lag and sleep disturbances, and more energy and alertness, compared to the group that took only the placebo. Surprisingly, the group that took melatonin all along reported a worse overall recovery from jet lag than the one that took the placebo at first. [Petrie]

High-dose melatonin is being investigated as a cancer treatment, both alone and in combination with other agents. In a study of 50 patients with brain metastases, 20 mgs of melatonin a day (plus supportive care) significantly increased survival time and slowed or stopped the growth of the metastases in the brain, as compared to supportive care alone. [Lissoni] *(Supportive care* aims merely to alleviate symptoms, not to cure the underlying ailment.) Melatonin may also enhance the effectiveness of cytokines (antitumor substances produced by the body's cells; interferon is an example), while decreasing their toxicity. [Brackowski]

Although currently available over the counter, melatonin is a powerful hormone that has a pronounced effect on reproductive hormones. In the 1970s, there was a brief flurry of interest in a method of contraception called *lunaception*. The theory—which has never been scientifically verified, as far as I know—is that if a woman sleeps outside under the light of the moon, her menstrual cycle synchronizes with the moon's cycle, making it easy to predict the date of ovulation and thus to avoid unprotected sex around that time. (This can be simulated indoors by sleeping in total darkness for most of the month, then with a dim lamp on in the room for three days a month.) The fact that melatonin affects the secretion of reproductive hormones probably accounts for whatever success lunaception enjoys.

There's no information available about long-term effects of taking melatonin every night, but occasional use is probably harmless. For those who want to stimulate their natural melatonin, there's certainly no harm in attempting to increase melatonin levels by sleeping in a completely dark room or using a sleep mask.

Ozone therapy

Ozone is a toxic gas that's a major component of smog. A reactive form of oxygen, it creates free radicals—in other words, it's an oxidizing agent and does just the opposite of what antioxidant vitamins do. But while oxidation is bad when it happens to healthy cells in your body, it's good when it happens to harmful foreign organisms.

Ozone inactivates many bacteria and viruses. That's why it's used for sewage treatment and water purification in this country, [Wells] and to treat tumors, fungal infections and acute and chronic viral infections in Europe. [Bocci] There's even some intriguing evidence that ozone is more toxic to cancer cells than to normal cells. [Sweet]

(Ozone also kills the HIV virus. But note that HIV is famously easy to kill, and that lots of substances that kill it *in vitro* aren't safe to use *in vivo*.)

While a small dose of ozone appears to enhance immune response, a larger dose can inhibit this same response. [Bocci, Paulesu] When inhaled, ozone can cause lung damage and injury to enzyme systems, red blood cells and the endocrine (hormonal) system. [Mehlman]

Therapeutic ozone is usually administered via a process called *autohemotherapy*, in which blood is removed from a patient, treated with ozone and then infused back into the patient. While this doesn't involve inhalation, there are many unknowns about long-term effects. Because ozone is quite toxic, effective only in a narrow range, and an accepted therapy only in other countries, I consider it to be closer to an unapproved drug than to an alternative therapy.

T'ai Chi

Sometimes called a moving meditation, T'ai Chi is a Chinese blend of exercise and energy work. Its arm movements are slow, circular, continuous, smooth and controlled, and weight is shifted regularly from one foot to the other. Groups of people concentrating on these rhythmical, dance-like movements are a common early-morning sight in parks in China, and T'ai Chi is now taught in many areas of the United States as well.

T'ai Chi may provide the health benefits of more strenuous exercise without straining the muscles or the heart. One study found that T'ai Chi increased breathing efficiency without stressing the cardiovascular system. [Brown]

Balance is important in preventing falls in the elderly. Nine healthy elderly Chinese T'ai Chi practitioners were compared with nine primarily sedentary but otherwise matched nonpractitioners on five balance measures. In three out of five of the tests, the T'ai Chi practitioners outperformed nonpractitioners.

The problem with this study is that it wasn't controlled for other types of exercise. Since the people who didn't do T'ai Chi were largely sedentary, the study may simply show the difference between out-of-shape people and relatively fit people. [Tse]

This seems to be borne out by another study that looked at how T'ai Chi affects recovery from stress. Ninety-six T'ai Chi practitioners were subjected to mental stress (doing arithmetic and other difficult mental tests under time pressure in a noisy environment) and, at another time, emotional stress (watching a film called *Horrible Experiences: a True Story*, specially edited to maximize horribleness). Measurements of stress hormones and mood disturbance scores validated the stress-producing effect of these sessions.

After each session, participants were divided into four groups: T'ai Chi, brisk walking, meditation or reading, each of which was practiced for an hour. The heart rate and blood pressure of the T'ai Chi practitioners was equivalent to the walkers. Once expectation was controlled for (T'ai Chi practitioners expected T'ai Chi to help them more), all of the four groups improved their mood and lowered their levels of stress hormones equally. [Jin]

SOURCES FOR REFERRALS

If some of the therapies described in this book sound useful to you, you'll want to know how to contact people who practice them. Here's a list of organizations that can make such referrals:

American Association of Naturopathic Physicians
2366 Eastlake Ave East, Ste 322, Seattle WA 98102
206 323 7610; fax: 206 323 7612
Professional association. Directory of members and brochure on naturopathy (which includes information on schools) available for $5 (check, money order or Visa/MasterCard).

Association for Applied Psychophysiology and Biofeedback
10200 West 44th Ave, Ste 304, Wheat Ridge CO 80033
303 422 8436; fax: 303 422 8894
Professional association; will refer to state associations. Information pamphlet available for a SASE.*

Biofeedback Certification Institute of America
10200 West 44th Ave, Ste 304, Wheat Ridge CO 80033
303 422 8894; fax: 303 422 8894
Certification agency. Referrals to certified practitioners in your area available for a SASE.*

American Massage Therapy Association
820 Davis St, Ste 100, Evanston IL 60201
708 864 0123; fax: 708 864 1178
Professional organization of graduates of AMTA-approved schools and people who have passed an AMTA exam.

American Chiropractic Association
1701 Clarendon Blvd, Arlington VA 22209
800 986 4636 or 703 276 8800; fax: 703 243 2593
Professional organization. Provides referrals on request.

American Herbalists Guild
Box 1683, Soquel CA 95073; 408 438 1700
Professional association. Publishes directory of classes & seminars.

---

*SASE = self-addressed stamped envelope (use a #10 envelope)

American Holistic Medical Association
4101 Lake Boone Trail, Ste 201, Raleigh NC 27607
919 787 5181; fax: 919 787 4916
Professional association of medical doctors and osteopathic physicians who incorporate various alternative therapies into their practices. Referral directory: $5.

American Holistic Nurses Association
4101 Lake Boone Trail, Ste 201, Raleigh NC 27607
919 787 5181; fax: 919 787 4916
Professional association of nurses who use various alternative therapies.

American Osteopathic Association
142 East Ontario St, Chicago IL 60611
312 280 5800; fax: 312 280 3860
Professional organization. Provides referrals to state associations.

American Society of Clinical Hypnosis
2200 East Devon Ave, Ste 291, Des Plaines IL 60018
847 297 3317; fax: 847 297 7309
Members are medical doctors and dentists trained in hypnosis. Referrals in your area available for a SASE.*

The Feldenkrais Guild
524 Ellsworth St or Box 489, Albany OR 97321
800 775 2118 or 541 926 0981; fax: 541 926 0572
Maintains list of certified practitioners. Membership list and catalog available on request.

National Center for Homeopathy
801 North Fairfax St, Ste 306, Alexandria VA 22314
703 548 7790; fax: 703 548 7792
Maintains directory of homeopaths who are also licensed health-care practitioners. Directory and packet of information for $6 (check or money order). Also offers courses.

National Commission for the Certification of Acupuncturists
1424 16th St NW, Ste 501, Washington DC 20036
202 232 1404; fax: 202 462 6157
Administers national certification exam to acupuncturists. State listing of members: $3. National listing: $22.

REFERENCES

Introduction

Anderson W, O'Connor BB, MacGregor RR, Schwartz JS. Patient use and assessment of conventional and alternative therapies for HIV infection and AIDS. *AIDS* 1993; 7:561–66.

Coleman LM, Fowler LL, Williams ME. Use of unproven therapies by people with Alzheimer's disease. *Journal of the American Geriatric Society* 1995; 43:747–50.

Eisenberg DM, Kessler RC, Foster C, et al. Unconventional medicine in the United States: prevalence, costs, and patterns of use. *New England Journal of Medicine* 1993; 328:246–52.

Acupuncture

Ballegaard S, Meyer CN, Trojaborg W. Acupuncture in angina pectoris: does acupuncture have a specific effect? *Journal of Internal Medicine* 1991; 229:357–62.

Barsoum G, Perry EP, Fraser IA. Postoperative nausea is relieved by acupressure. *Journal of the Royal Society of Medicine* 1990; 83:86–89.

Brewington V, Smith M, Lipton D. Acupuncture as a detoxification treatment: an analysis of controlled research. *Journal of Substance Abuse Treatment* 1994; 11(4):289–307.

Bullock ML, Culliton PD, Olander RT. Controlled trial of acupuncture for severe recidivist alcoholism. *Lancet* 1989:1435–38.

Bullock ML, Umen AJ, Culliton PD, Olander RT. Acupuncture treatment of alcoholic recidivism: a pilot study. *Alcoholism: Clinical and Experimental Reaearch* 1987; 11:292–95.

Cahn AM, Carayon P, Hill C, Flamant R. Acupuncture in gastroscopy. *Lancet* 1978:182–83.

Carlsson J, Fahlcrantz A, Augustinsson LE. Muscle tenderness in tension headache treated with acupuncture or physiotherapy. *Cephalalgia* Jun 1990; 10(3):131–41.

Chow OKW, So SY, Lam WK, et al. Effect of acupuncture on exercise-induced asthma. *Lung* 1983; 161:321–26.

Christensen BV, Iuhl IU, Vilbek H et al. Acupuncture treatment of severe knee osteoarthrosis. A long-term study. *Acta Anaesthesiologica Scandanavica* Aug 1992; 36(6):519–25.

Christensen PA, Laursen LC, Taudorf E, et al. Acupuncture and bronchial asthma. *Allergy* 1984; 39:379–85.

Christensen PA, Noreng M, Andersen PE, Nielsen JW. Electroacupuncture and postoperative pain. *British Journal of Anaesthesia* 1989; 62:258–62.

Coan RM, Wong G, Coan PL. The acupuncture treatment of low back pain: a randomized controlled study. *American Journal of Chinese Medicine* 1980; 8:181–89.

Coan RM, Wong G, Coan PL. The acupuncture treatment of neck pain: a randomized controlled study. *American Journal of Chinese Medicine* 1982; 9:326–32.

De Aloysio D, Penacchioni P. Morning sickness control in early pregnancy by Neiguan point acupressure. *Obstetrics and Gynecology* 1992; 80:852–54.

Dowson DI, Lewith GT, Machin D. The effects of acupuncture versus placebo in the treatment of headache. *Pain* 1985; 21:35–42.

Dundee JW, Yang J, McMillan C. Non-invasive stimulation of the P-6 (Neiguan) antiemetic acupuncture point in cancer chemotherapy. *Journal of the Royal Society of Medicine* Apr 1991; 84(4):210–12.

Dunn PA, App M, Rogers D, Halford K. Transcutaneous electrical nerve stimulation at acupuncture points in the induction of uterine contractions. *Obstetrics and Gynecology* 1989; 73:286–90.

Ehrlich D and Haber P. Influence of acupuncture on physical performance capacity and haemodynamic parameters. *International Journal of Sports Medicine* 1992; 13:486–91.

Fung KP, Chow OKW, So SY. Attenuation of exercise-induced asthma by acupuncture. *Lancet* 1986:1419–22.

Gaw AC, Chang LW, Shaw LC. Efficacy of acupuncture on osteoarthritic pain. *New England Journal of Medicine* 1975; 293:375–78.

Helms JM. Acupuncture for the management of primary dysmenorrhea. *Obstetrics and Gynecology* 1987; 69:51–56.

Hu H-H, Chung C, Liu TJ, et al. A randomized controlled trial on the treatment for acute partial ischemic stroke with acupuncture. *Neuroepidemiology* 1993; 12:106–13.

Hyde E. Acupressure therapy for morning sickness: a controlled clinical trial. *Journal of Nurse-Midwifery* 1989; 34 (4):171–78.

Jobst K, McPherson K, Brown V, et al. Controlled trial of acupuncture for disabling breathlessness. *Lancet* 1986:1416–19.

Kent GP, Brondum J, Keenlyside RA, et al. A large outbreak of acupuncture-associated hepatitis B. *American Journal of Epidemiology* 1988; 127(3):591–98.

Kleijnen J, ter Riet G, Knipschild P. Acupuncture and asthma: a review of controlled trials. *Thorax* 1991; 46:799–802.

Kroening RJ, Oleson TD. Rapid narcotic detoxification in chronic pain patients treated with auricular electroacupuncture and naloxone. *The International Journal of the Addictions* 1985; 20(9):1347–60.

Lee YH, Lee WC, Chen MT, et al. Acupuncture in the treatment of renal colic. *Journal of Urology* Jan 1992; 147(1):16–18.

Lewith GT, Field J, Machin D. Acupuncture compared with placebo in post-herpetic pain. *Pain* 1983; 17:361–68.

Lytle CD. *An overview of acupuncture.* Center for Devices and Radiological Health, Food and Drug Administration, 1993, Public Health Service, Rockville, MD.

Man P, Chuang M. Acupuncture in methadone withdrawal. *International Journal of the Addictions* 1980; 15:921–26.

NCCA. Safety record of acupuncture. National Commission for the Certification of Acupuncturists, Feb 1993. Available from NCCA, 1424 16th St, Suite 501, Washington DC 20036.

Newmeyer T, Johnson G, Klot S. Acupuncture as a detoxification modality. *Journal of Psychoactive Drugs* 1984; 16:241–61.

Patel M, Gutzwiller F, Paccaud F, Marazzi A. A meta-analysis of acupuncture for chronic pain. *International Journal of Epidemiology* Dec 1989; 18(4):900–906.

Richter A, Herlitz J, Hjalmarson A. Effect of acupuncture in patients with angina pectoris. *European Heart Journal* Feb 1991; 12(2)175–78.

Tashkin DP, Bresler DE, Kroening RJ, et al. Comparison of real and simulated acupuncture and isoproterenol in methacholine-induced asthma. *Annals of Allergy* 1977; 39(6):379–87.

Tashkin DP, Kroening RJ, Bresler DE, et al. A controlled trial of real and simulated acupuncture in the management of chronic asthma. *Journal of Allergy and Clinical Immunology* 1985; 76:855–64.

203

Tavola T, Gala C, Conte G, Invernizzi G. Traditional Chinese acupuncture in tension-type headache: a controlled study. *Pain* Mar 1992; 48(3):325–29.

ter Riet G, Kleijnen J, Knipschild P. Acupuncture and chronic pain: a criteria-based meta-analysis. *Journal of Clinical Epidemiology* 1990; 43(11):1191–99.

Vincent CA. A controlled trial of the treatment of migraine by acupuncture. *Clinical Journal of Pain* Dec 1989; 5(4):305–12.

Vincent CA. The treatment of tension headache by acupuncture: a controlled single case design with time series analysis. *Journal of Psychosomatic Research* 1990; 34(5):553–61.

Warwick-Evans LA, Masters IJ, Redstone SB. A double-blind placebo controlled evaluation of acupressure in the treatment of motion sickness. *Aviation, Space, and Environmental Medicine* 1991; 62:776–78.

Washburn AM, Fullilove RE, Fullilive MT, et al. Acupuncture heroin detoxification: a single-blind clinical trial. *Journal of Substance Abuse Treatment* 1993; 10:345–51.

Yang LC, Jawan B, Chen CN, et al. Comparison of P6 acupoint injection with 50% glucose in water and intravenous droperidol for prevention of vomiting after gynecological laparoscopy. *Acta Anaesthesiologica Scandanavica* Feb 1993; 37(2):192–94.

Yentis SM, Bissonnette B. P6 acupuncture and postoperative vomiting after tonsillectomy in children. *British Journal of Anaesthesia* 1991; 67:779–80.

Ayurveda and yoga

Charles V, Charles SX. The use and efficacy of Azadirachta indica ADR ('Neem') and Curcuma longa ('Turmeric') in scabies: a pilot study. *Tropical and Geographical Medicine* 1992; 44:178–81.

Dash VB. *Fundamentals of Ayurvedic Medicine.* Konark Publishers Pvt Ltd, 1978, (7th revised edition 1989, reprinted 1992), A-149, Main Vikas Marg, Delhi 110092 India.

Devaraj TL. *The Panchakarma Treatment of Ayurveda.* Dhanvantari Oriental Publications, 1980 (reprinted 1986), 90 Sarvabhouma Colony, Chikalsandra, Subramanyapura Post, Bangalore, India.

Dwivedi C, Sharma H, Dobrowski S, Engineer FN. Inhibitory effects of Maharishi-4 and Maharishi-5 on microsomal lipid peroxidation. *Pharmacology, Biochemistry and Behavior* 1991; 39:649–52.

Goyeche JRM, Abo Y, Ikemi Y. Asthma: the yoga perspective. Part II: Yoga therapy in the treatment of asthma. *Journal of Asthma* 1982; 19(3):189–201.

Jacob A, Pandey M, Kapoor S, Saroja R. Effect of the Indian Gooseberry (Amla) on serum cholesterol levels in men aged 35–55 years. *European Journal of Clinical Nutrition* 1988; 42:939–44.

Jain SC, Rai L, Valecha A, et al. Effect of yoga training on exercise tolerance in adolescents with childhood asthma. *Journal of Asthma* 1991; 28(6):437–42.

Jain SC, Uppal A, Bhatnagar SOD, Tulukdar B. A study of response pattern of non-insulin-dependent diabetics to yoga therapy. *Diabetes Research and Clinical Practice* 1993; 19:69–74.

Klein AC, Sobel D. *Backache Relief.* New American Library, 1985, New York.

Klein R, Pilon D, Prosser S. Nasal airflow asymmetries and human performance. *Biological Psychology* 1986; 23:127–37.

Lad V. *Ayurveda: the science of self-healing.* Lotus Press, 1984, Santa Fe NM.

Niwa Y. Effect of Maharishi-4 and Maharishi-5 on inflammatory mediators with special reference to their free radical scavenging effect. *Indian Journal of Clinical Practice* 1991; 1:23–27.

Patel CH. Yoga and biofeedback in the management of hypertension. *Lancet* 1973:1053–55.

Salerno JW, Smith DE. The use of sesame oil and other vegetable oils in the inhibition of human colon cancer growth in vitro. *Anticancer Research* 1991; 11:209–16.

Shanahoff-Khalsa DS, Boyle MR, Buebel ME. The effects of unilateral forced nostril breathing on cognition. *International Journal of Neuroscience* 1991; 57:239–49.

Sharma HM, Dwivedi C, Satter BC, et al. Antineoplastic properties of Maharishi-4 against DMBA-induced mammary tumors in rats. *Pharmacology Biochemistry and Behavior* 1990; 35:767–73.

Sharma HM, Feng Y, Panganamala RV. Maharishi Amrit Kalash (MAK) prevents human platelet aggregation. *Clinica E Terapia Cardiovascolare* 1989; 8:227–30.

Sharma HM, Triguna BD, Chopra D. Maharishi Ayur-Veda: Modern insights into ancient medicine. *Journal of the American Medical Association* 1991; 265:2633–37.

Skolnick A. Maharishi Ayur-Veda: Guru's marketing scheme promises the world eternal 'perfect health'. *Journal of the American Medical Association* 1991; 266:1741–50.

Thyagarajan SP, Subramanian S, Thirunalasundari T, et al. Effect of Phyllanthus amarus on chronic carriers of hepatitis B virus. *Lancet* 1988:764–66.

Unander DW, Webster GL, Blumberg BS. Usage and bioassays in phyllanthus (Euphorbiacaea) IV clustering of antiviral uses and other effects. *Journal of Ethnopharmacology* 1995; 45(1):1–18.

Werntz DA, Bickford RG, Shanahoff-Khalsa D. Selective hemispheric stimulation by unilateral forced nostril breathing. *Human Neurobiology* 1987; 6:165–71.

Wood C. Mood change and perceptions of vitality: a comparison of the effects of relaxation, visualization and yoga. *Journal of the Royal Society of Medicine* 1993; 86(5):254–58.

Biofeedback

Andrasik F. Psychologic and behavioral aspects of chronic headache. *Neurologic Clinics* 1990; 8(4):961–76.

Blanchard EB, Andrasik F. Biofeedback treatment of vascular headache. In *Biofeedback: Studies in Clinical Efficacy,* edited by JP Hatch, JG Fisher, JD Rugh. Plenum, 1987, New York:1–79.

Brocklehurst JC. Management of anal incontinence. *Clinical Gastroenterology* 1975; 4:479–87.

Bruhn P, Olesen J, Melgaard B. Controlled trial of EMG feedback in muscle contraction headache. *Annals of Neurology* 1979; 6:34–36.

Burns PA, Pranikoff K, Nochajski TH, et al. Treatment of stress incontinence with pelvic floor exercises and biofeedback. *Journal of the American Geriatrics Society* 1990; 38:341–44. Also, A comparison of effectiveness of biofeedback and pelvic muscle exercise treatment of stress incontinence in older community-dwelling women. *Journal of Gerontology* 1993; 48(4):M167–M174.

Cardozo LD, Abrams PD, Stanton SL, Fenely RC. Idiopathic bladder instability treated by biofeedback. *British Journal of Urology* 1978; 50(7):521–23.

Chiarioni G, Scattolini C, Bonfante F, Vantini I. Liquid stool incontinence with severe urgency: anorectal function and effective biofeedback treatment. *Gut* 1993; 34:1576–80.

Diokno AC, Brock BM, Brown MB, Herzog AR. Prevalence of urinary incontinence and other urological symptoms in the noninstitutionalized elderly. *Journal of Urology* 1986; 136(5):1022–25.

Glasgow MS, Engel BT. Biofeedback and relaxation therapy. In *Biofeedback: Studies in Clinical Efficacy,* edited by JP Hatch, JG Fisher, JD Rugh. Plenum, 1987, New York:81–122.

Jahanshahi M, Sartory G, Marsden CD. EMG biofeedback treatment of torticollis: a controlled outcome study. *Biofeedback and Self-Regulation* 1991; 16(4):413–48.

Latham PM. Diseases of the heart. Lect. XXXVIII. Quoted in *Familiar Medical Quotations*, edited by MB Strauss, Little, Brown & Co, 1968, Boston:41.

Marzuk PM. Biofeedback for gastrointestinal disorders: a review of the literature. *Annals of Internal Medicine* 1985; 103:240–44.

McIntosh LJ, Frahm JD, Mallett VT, Richardson DA. Pelvic floor rehabilitation in the treatment of incontinence. *Journal of Reproductive Medicine* 1993; 38(9):662–65.

Peniston EG, Kulkosky PJ. Alpha-theta brainwave neuro-feedback therapy for Vietnam veterans with combat-related post-traumatic stress disorder. *Medical Psychotherapy* 1991; 4:47–60.

Peniston EG, Kulkosky PJ. Alpha-theta brainwave training and beta-endorphin levels in alcoholics. *Alcoholism: Clinical and Experimental Research* 1989; 13(2):271–79.

Podoshin L, Ben-David Y, Fradis M, et al. Idiopathic subjective tinnitus treated by biofeedback, acupuncture and drug therapy. *Ear, Nose and Throat Journal* 1991; 70(5):284–89.

Rice BI, Schindler JV. Effect of thermal biofeedback-assisted relaxation training on blood circulation in the lower extremities of a population with diabetes. *Diabetes Care* Jul 1992; 15(7):853–58.

Ross B, Nedzelski JM, McLean A. Efficacy of feedback training in long-standing facial nerve paresis. *Laryngoscope* 1991; 101(7,Part 1):744–50.

Schleenbaker RE, Mainous III, AG. Electromyographic biofeedback for neuromuscular reeducation in the hemiplegic stroke patient: a meta-analysis. *Archives of Physical Medicine and Rehabilitation* 1993; 74(12):1301–04.

Susset J, Galea G, Manbeck K, Susset A. A predictive score index for the outcome of associated biofeedback and vaginal electrical stimulation in the treatment of female incontinence. *Journal of Urology* 1995; 153(5):1461–66.

Whitehead WE, Schuster MM. Fecal incontinence. In *Gastrointestinal disorders: behavioral and physiological basis for treatment,* edited by RS Surwit, RB Williams Jr, D Shapiro. Academic Press, 1985, Orlando:229–75.

Chiropractic, etc.

ABCA. American Black Chiropractors Association, 17301 W Eight Mile Rd, Detroit MI 48235.

ACA. American Chiropractic Association, 1701 Clarendon Blvd, Arlington VA 22209.

AOA. American Osteopathic Association, 142 East Ontario St, Chicago IL 60611.

Anderson R, Meeker WC, Wirick BE, et al. A meta-analysis of clinical trials of spinal manipulation. *Journal of Manipulative and Physiological Therapeutics* 1992; 15(3):181–94.

Bergquist-Ullmann M, Larsson U. Acute low back pain in industry. *Acta Orthopaedica Scandanavica* 1977; 170: 1–117.

Bigos SJ, Bowyer OR, Braen GR, et al. *Acute Low Back Problems in Adults, Clinical Practice Guideline #14* 1994. US Department of Health and Human Services, PHS Agency for Health Care Policy and Research, Rockville MD.

Cherkin DC and MacCornack FA. Patient evaluations of low back pain care from family physicians and chiropractors. *Western Journal of Medicine* 1989; 150:351–55.

Chrisman D, Mittnacht A, Snook GA. A study of the results following rotatory manipulation in the lumbar intervertebral-disc syndrome. *Journal of Bone and Joint Surgery* 1964; 46:517–24.

Coxhead CE, Meade TW, Inskip H, et al. Multicentre trial of physiotherapy in the management of sciatic symptoms. *Lancet* 1981:1065–68.

Coyer AB and Curwen IHM. Low back pain treated by manipulation: a controlled series. *British Medical Journal* 1955; 1:705–07.

Doran ML, Newell DJ. Manipulation in treatment of low back pain: a multicentre study. *British Medical Journal* 1975; 2:161–64.

Eisenberg DM, Kessler RC, Foster C, et al. Unconventional medicine in the United States: prevalence, costs, and patterns of use. *New England Journal of Medicine* 1993; 328:246–52.

Glover JR, Morris JG, Khosla T. Back pain: a randomized clinical trial of rotational manipulation of the trunk. *British Journal of Industrial Medicine* 1974; 31:59–64.

Godfrey CM, Morgan PP, Schatzker J. A randomized trial of manipulation for low back pain in a medical setting. *Spine* 1984; 9(3):301–04.

Hadler NM, Curtis P, Gillings DB, Stinett S. A benefit of spinal manipulation as adjunctive therapy for low back pain: a stratified controlled trial. *Spine* 1987; 12:703–06.

Jensen MC, Brant-Zawadski MN, Obuchowski N, et al. Magnetic resonance imaging of the lumbar spine in people without back pain. *New England Journal of Medicine* 1994; 331(2):69–73.

Kane RL, Olsen D, Leymaster C, et al. Manipulating the patient: a comparison of the effectiveness of physician and chiropractor care. *Lancet* 1974:1333–36.

Klougart N, Nilsson N, Jacobsen J. Infantile colic treated by chiropractors: a prospective study of 316 cases. *Journal of Manipulative and Physiological Therapeutics* 1989; 12(4):281–88.

Koes BW, Assendelft WJJ, van der Heijden GJMG, et al. Spinal manipulation and mobilisation for back and neck pain: a blinded review. *British Medical Journal* 1991; 303:1298–1303.

Koes BW, Bouter LM, van Mameren H, et al. A blinded randomized clinical trial of manual therapy and physiotherapy for chronic back and neck complaints: physical therapy measures. *Journal of Manipulative and Physiological Therapeutics* 1992; 15(1):16–23.

Kokjohn K, Schmid DM, Triano JJ, Brennan PC. The effects of spinal manipulation on pain and prostaglandin levels in women with primary dysmenorrhea. *Journal of Manipulative and Physiological Therapeutics* 1992; 15(5):279–85.

Ladermann JP. Accidents of spinal manipulations. *Annals of the Swiss Chiropractors Association* 1981; 7:161–208.

MacDonald RS and Bell, CMJ. An open controlled assessment of osteopathic manipulation in nonspecific low-back pain. *Spine* 1990; 15(5):364–70.

Mathews JA, Mills, SB, Jenkins VM, et al. Back pain and sciatica: controlled trials of manipulation, traction, sclerosant and epidural injections. *British Journal of Rheumatology* 1987; 26:416–23.

Meade TW, Dyer S, Browne W, et al. Low back pain of mechanical origin: randomized comparison of chiropractic and hospital outpatient treatment. *British Medical Journal* 1990; 300:1431–37.

Moore JS. *Chiropractic in America.* Johns Hopkins University Press, 1993, Baltimore MD:16.

Moore. 104.

Moore. 105–108.

Moore. 111–15.

Moore. 127.

Moore. 128.

Moore. 129–30.

Moore. 131–37.

Morgan JP, Dickey JL, Hunt HH, Hudgins PM. A controlled trial of spinal manipulation in the management of hypertension. *Journal of the American Osteopathic Association* 1985; 85:308–13.

Nielsen NH, Bronfort G, Bendix T, et al. Chronic asthma and chiropractic spinal manipulation: a randomized clinical trial. *Clinical and Experimental Allergy* 1995; 25:80–88.

Ottenbacher K and Difabio RP. Efficacy of spinal manipulation/manipulation therapy: a meta-analysis. *Spine* 1985; 10:833–37.

Parker GB, Tupling H, Pryor DS. A controlled trial of cervical manipulation for migraine. *Australia and New Zealand Journal of Medicine* 1978; 8:589–93.

Raftis KL, Warfield CA. Spinal manipulation for back pain. *Hospital Practice* 1989; Mar 15:89–108.

Reed WR, Beavers S, Reddy SK, Kern G. Chiropractic management of primary nocturnal enuresis. *Journal of Manipulative and Physiological Therapeutics* 1994; 17:596–600.

Shekelle PG, Adams AH, Chassin MR, et al. Spinal manipulation for low-back pain. *Annals of Internal Medicine* 1992; 117(7):590–98.

Shekelle PG, Brook RH. A community based study of the use of chiropractic services. *American Journal of Public Health* 1991; 81(4):439–42.

Sims-Williams H, Jayson MIV, Young SMS, et al. Controlled trial of mobilisation and manipulation for low back pain: hospital patients. *British Medical Journal* 1979; 2:1318–20.

Sims-Williams H, Jayson MIV, Young SMS, et al. Controlled trial of mobilisation and manipulation for patients with low back pain in general practice. *British Medical Journal* 1978; 2:1338–40.

Thomason PR, Fisher BL, Carpenter BL, Fike GL. Effectiveness of spinal manipulative therapy in treatment of primary dysmenorrhea: a pilot study. *Journal of Manipulative and Physiological Therapeutics* 1979; 2(3):140–45.

Von Kuster T Jr. *Chiropractic health care: a national study of cost of education, service, utilization, number of practicing doctors of chiropractic and other key policy issues.* Foundation for the advancement of chiropractic tenets and science, 1980, Washington DC.

Walsh MR. *Doctors Wanted: No Women Need Apply.* Yale University Press, 1977, New Haven and London:224.

Wilson JN, Ilfield FW. Manipulation of the herniated disc. *American Journal of Surgery* 1952; 83:173–75.

Dietary supplements

ABCPSG. Alpha-tocopherol, beta-carotene cancer prevention study group. The effect of vitamin E and beta-carotene on the incidence of lung cancer and other cancers in male smokers. *New England Journal of Medicine* 1994; 330:1029–35.

Adlercreutz H, Honjo H, Higashi A, et al. Urinary excretion of lignans and isoflavonoid phytoestrogens in Japanese men and women consuming a traditional Japanese diet. *American Journal of Clinical Nutrition* 1991; 54:1093–1100.

Adlercreutz H, Hamalainen E, Gorbach S, Goldin B. Dietary phytoestrogens and the menopause in Japan. *Lancet* 1992; 339:1233.

Adlercreutz H. Isoflavonoids and lignans in man: history, presence in food, and epidemiology in relation to cancer. Presented at the conference *Dietary Phytoestrogens: cancer cause or prevention?,* sponsored by the National Cancer Institute. Herndon VA, Sept. 21–23, 1994.

Alderman JD, Pasternak RC, Sacks FM, et al. Effect of a modified, well-tolerated niacin regimen on serum total cholesterol, high-density lipoprotein cholesterol and the cholesterol to high-density cholesterol ratio. *American Journal of Cardiology* 1989; 64:725–29.

Anderson JW, Johnstone BM, Cook-Newell ME. Meta-analysis of the effects of soy protein intake on serum lipids. *New England Journal of Medicine* 1995; 333:276-282.

Anibarro B, Caballero T, Garcia-Ara C, et al. Asthma with sulfite intolerance in children: a blocking study with cyanocobalamin. *Journal of Allergy and Clinical Immunology* 1992; 90:103–9.

Ascherio A, Willett WC. Are body iron stores related to the risk of coronary heart disease? *New England Journal of Medicine* 1994; 330:1152–53.

Bartels GL, Remme WJ, Pillay M, et al. Effects of l-propionylcarnitine on ischemia-induced myocardial dysfunction in men with angina pectoris. *American Journal of Cardiology* 1994; 74:125–30.

Belch JJF, Ansell D, Madhok R, et al. Effects of altering dietary essential fatty acids on requirements for non-steroidal anti-inflammatory drugs in patients with rheumatoid arthritis: a double-blind placebo-controlled trial. *Annals of the Rheumatic Diseases* 1988; 47:96–104.

Belizan JM, Villar J, Gonzalez L, et al. Calcium supplementation to prevent hypertensive disorders of pregnancy. *New England Journal of Medicine* 1991; 325:1399–1405.

Bentivoglio G, Melica F, Cristoforoni P. Folinic acid in the treatment of human male infertility. *Fertility and Sterility* 1993; 60:698–701.

Berth-Jones J, Graham-Brown RAC. Placebo-controlled trial of essential fatty acid supplementation in atopic dermatitis. *Lancet* 1993; 341:1557–60.

Bielory L, Gandhi R. Asthma and vitamin C. *Annals of Allergy* 1994; 73:89–96.

Bittiner SB, Cartwright I, Tucker WFG, Bleehan SS. A double-blind, random-ized, placebo-controlled trial of fish oil in psoriasis. *Lancet* 1988:378–80.

Bjorneboe A, Soyland E, Bjorneboe G-EA, et al. Effect of dietary supplementa-tion with eicasopentaenoic acid in the treatment of atopic dermatitis. *British Journal of Dermatology* 1987; 117:463–69.

Block G, Menkes M. Ascorbic acid in cancer prevention. In *Nutrition and Cancer Prevention: investigating the role of micronutrients*, edited by TE Moon, MS Micozzi. Marcel Dekker, 1989, New York and Basel:243–73.

Blot WJ, Li J-Y, Taylor P, et al. Nutrition intervention trials in Linxian, China: supplementation with specific vitamin/mineral combinations, cancer incidence, and disease-specific mortality in the general population. *Journal of the National Cancer Institute* 1993; 85:1483–92.

Bourgoin BP, Evans DR, Cornett JR, et al. Lead content in 70 brands of dietary calcium supplements. *American Journal of Public Health* 1993; 83:1155–60.

Brevetti G, Chiariello M, Ferulano G, et al. Increases in walking distance in patients with peripheral vascular disease treated with L-carnitine: a double-blind, cross-over study. *Circulation* 1988; 77(4):767–73.

Brodsky MA, Orlov MV, Capparelli EV et al. Magnesium therapy in new-onset atrial fibrillation. *American Journal of Cardiology* 1994;73:1227–29.

Butterworth CE and Tamura T. Folic acid safety and toxicity: a brief review. *American Journal of Clinical Nutrition* 1989; 50:353–58.

Butterworth CE, Hatch KD, Macaluso M, et al. Folate deficiency and cervical dysplasia. *Journal of the American Medical Association* 1992; 267(4):528–33.

Carlson SE, Wertkman SH, Rhodes PG, Tolley EA. Visual-acuity development in healthy preterm infants; effect of marine-oil supplementation. *American Journal of Clinical Nutrition* 1993; 58:35–42.

Chandra RK. Effect of vitamin and trace-element supplementation on immune responses and infections in elderly subjects. *Lancet* 1992; 340:1124–27.

Chello M, Mastroroberto P, Romano R, et al. Protection by coenzyme Q10 from myocardial reperfusion injury during coronary artery bypass grafting. *Annals of Thoracic Surgery* 1994; 58:1427–32.

Cherchi A, Lai C, Angelino F, et al. Effects of L-carnitine on exercise tolerance in chronic stable angina; a multicenter, double-blind, randomized, placebo-controlled crossover study. *International Journal of Clinical Pharmacology, Therapy, and Toxicology* 1985; 23(10):569–72.

Chouinard G, Young SN, Bradwejn J, Annable L. Tryptophan in the treatment of depression and mania. *Advances in Biological Psychiatry* 1983; 10:47–66.

Christensen AN, Achor RWP, Berge KG, Mason HL. Nicotinic acid treatment of hypercholesterolemia. *Journal of the American Medical Association* 1961; 177:546–50.

Cleland LG, French JK, Betts WH, et al. Clinical and biochemical effects of dietary fish oil supplements in rheumatoid arthritis. *Journal of Rheumatology* 1988; 15:1471–75.

Clemmensen OJ, Siggaard-Andersen, Worm AM, et al. Psoriatic arthritis treated with oral zinc sulphate. *British Journal of Dermatology* 1980; 103:411–15.

Combs GF. Selenium. In *Nutrition and Cancer Prevention: investigating the role of micronutrients*, edited by TE Moon, MS Micozzi. Marcel Dekker, 1989, New York and Basel:389–420.

Coull BM, Malinow MR, Beamer N, et al. Elevated plasma homocysteine concentration as a possible independent risk factor for stroke. *Stroke* 1990; 21:572–76.

Cutler JA, Brittain E. Calcium and blood pressure: an epidemiological perspective. *American Journal of Hypertension* 1990; 3:137S–146S.

Darlington LG, Ramsey NW. Review of dietary therapy for rheumatoid arthritis. *British Journal of Rheumatology* 1993; 32:507–14.

Davini P, Bigalli A, Lamanna F, Boem A. Controlled study on L-carnitine therapeutic efficacy in post-infarction. *Drugs Under Experimental & Clinical Research* 1992; 18(8):355–64.

DiGiovanna JJ, Blank H. Failure of lysine in frequently recurrent herpes simplex infection. *Archives of Dermatology* 1984; 120:48–51.

Donadio JV, Bergstralh EJ, Offord KP, et al. A controlled trial of fish oil in IgA nephropathy. *New England Journal of Medicine* 1994; 331:1194–99.

Douglas RM, Miles HB, Moore BW, et al. Failure of effervescent zinc acetate lozenges to alter the course of upper respiratory tract infections in Australian adults. *Antimicrobial Agents and Chemotherapy* 1987; 31:1263–65.

Dwyer JT, Goldin BR, Saul N, et al. Tofu and soy drinks contain phytoestrogens. *Journal of the American Dietetic Association* 1994; 94:739-743.

Ebiling PR, Sandgren ME, Di Magno EP, et al. Evidence of an age-related decrease in intestinal responsiveness to vitamin D: relationship between serum 1,25 dihydroxyvitamin D and intestinal vitamin D receptor concentration in normal women. *Journal of Clinical Endocrinology and Metabolism* 1992; 75:176–82.

Eby GA, Davis DR, Halcomb WH. Reduction in duration of common colds by zinc gluconate lozenges in a double-blind study. *Antimicrobial Agents and Chemotherapy* 1984; 25:20–24.

Edwards B. *America's Favorite Drug: Coffee and Your Health.* Odonian 1992:47–49.

EM. *Emergency Medicine.*Vitamins with a vengeance (anonymous), 1992; Mar 15:274–82.

England MR, Gordon G, Salem M, Chernow B. Magnesium administration and dysrhythmias after cardiac surgery. *Journal of the American Medical Association* 1992; 268:2395–2402.

Faccinetti F, Sances G, Borella P, et al. Magnesium prophylaxis of menstrual migraine: effects on intracellular magnesium. *Headache* 1991; 321:298–301.

Farr BM, Conner EM, Betts RF, et al. Two randomized controlled trials of zinc gluconate lozenge therapy of experimentally induced rhinovirus colds. *Antimicrobial Agents and Chemotherapy* 1987; 31(8):1183–87.

Fawzi WW, Chalmers TC, Herrera G, Mosteller F. Vitamin A supplementation and child mortality. *Journal of the American Medical Association* 1993; 269:898–903.

Gallai V, Sarchielli P, Morucci P, Abritti G. Red blood cell magnesium levels in migraine patients. *Cephalalgia* 1993; 13:94–98.

Gapinski JP, VanRuiswyk JVV, Heudebert GR, Schectman GS. Preventing restenosis with fish oils following coronary angioplasty. *Archives of Internal Medicine* 1993; 153:1595–1601.

Garland FC, Garland CF, Gorham ED, Young JF. Geographic variation in breast cancer mortality in the United States: a hypothesis involving exposure to solar radiation. *Preventive Medicine* 1990; 19:614–22.

Ghent WR, Eskin BA, Low DA, Hill LP. Iodine replacement in fibrocystic disease of the breast. *Canadian Journal of Surgery* 1993; 36:453–60.

Giovannucci E, Stampfer MJ, Colditz GA, et al. Folate, methionine, and alcohol intake and risk of colorectal adenoma. *Journal of the National Cancer Institute* 1993; 85(11):875–84.

Godfrey JC, Sloane BC, Smith DS, et al. Zinc gluconate and the common cold: a controlled clinical study. *Journal of International Medical Research* 1992; 20:234–46.

Gould KL, Ornish D, Kirkeeide R, et al. Improved stenosis geometry by quantitative coronary arteriography after vigorous risk factor modification. *American Journal of Cardiology* 1992; 69(9):845–53.

Grant ECG. Food allergies and migraine. *Lancet* 1979:966–68.

Griffith RS, Norins AL, Kagan C. A multicentered study of lysine therapy in herpes simplex infection. *Dermatologica* 1977; 156:257–67.

Grudley G, Mclaughlin JK, Block G, et al. Vitamin supplement use and reduced risk of oral and pharyngeal cancer. *American Journal of Epidemiology* 1992; 135:1083–92.

Hankinson SE, Stampfer MJ, Seddon JM, et al. Nutrient intake and cataract extraction in women: a prospective study. *British Medical Journal* 1992; 305:335–39.

Hatton DC, McCarron DA. Dietary calcium and blood pressure in experimental models of hypertension: a review. *Hypertension* 1994; 23(4):513–26.

Hertog MG, Kromhout D, Aravanis C, et al. Flavonoid intake and long-term risk of coronary heart disease and cancer in the seven countries study. *Archives of Internal Medicine* 1995; 155(4):381–86.

Hertog MGL, Feskens JM, Hollman PCH, et al. Dietary antioxidant flavonoids and risk of coronary heart disease: the Zutphen elderly study. *Lancet* 1993; 342:1007–11.

Higgins GL. Magnesium medicine comes of age. *Emergency Medicine* Feb 1991:83–95.

Horner SM. Efficacy of intravenous magnesium in acute myocardial infarction in reducing arrhythmias and mortality. *Circulation* 1992; 86:774–79.

Hunter DJ, Manson JE, Colditz GA, et al. A prospective study of the intake of vitamins C, E, and A and the risk of breast cancer. *New England Journal of Medicine* 1993; 329:234–40.

Idjradinata P, Watkins WE, Pollitt E. Adverse effect of iron supplementation on weight gain of iron-replete young children. *Lancet* 1994; 343:1252–54.

Israelsson B, Brattstrom LE, Hultberg BL. Homocysteine and myocardial infarction. *Atherosclerosis* 1988; 71:227–33.

Jancin B. *Family Practice News* 1994; Mar 1:10.

Jewett DL, Fein G, Greenberg MH. A double-blind study of symptom provocation to determine food sensitivity. *New England Journal of Medicine* 1990; 323(7): 429–33.

Jones VA, Dickinson RJ, Workman E, et al. Crohn's disease: maintenance of remission with diet. *Lancet* 1985:177–80.

Kagan C. Lysine therapy for herpes simplex. *Lancet* 1974:137.

Kamikawa T, Kobayashi A, Yamashita T, et al. Effects of coenzyme Q10 on exercise tolerance in chronic stable angina pectoris. *American Journal of Cardiology* 1985; 56:247–51.

Kardinaal AFM, Kok FJ, Ringstad J, et al. Antioxidants in adipose tissue and risk of myocardial infarction: the Euramic study. *Lancet* 1993; 342:1379–84.

Khaw K-T, Barrett-Connor E. Dietary potassium and stroke-related mortality. *New England Journal of Medicine* 1987; 316:235–40.

Kjeldsen-Kragh J, Haugen M, Borchgrevink CF, et al. Controlled trial of fasting and one-year vegetarian diet in rheumatoid arthritis. *Lancet* 1991; 338:899–902.

Kremer JM, Michalek AV, Lininger L, et al. Effects of manipulation of dietary fatty acids on clinical manifestations of rheumatoid arthritis. *Lancet* 1985:184–87.

Kunz B, Ring J, Braun-Falco O. Eicasopentanoic acid (EPA) treatment in atopic eczema. *Journal of Allergy and Clinical Immunology* 1989; 83:196.

Lakka TA, Nyyssonen K, Salonen JT. Higher levels of conditioning leisure time physical activity are associated with reduced levels of stored iron in Finnish men. *American Journal of Epidemiology* 1994; 140:148–60.

Lamm DL, Riggs DR, Shriver JS, et al. Megadose vitamins in bladder cancer: a double-blind clinical trial. *Journal of Urology* 1994; 151:21–26.

Lassus A, Dahlgren AL, Halpern MJ, et al. Effects of dietary supplementation with polyunsaturated ethyl ester lipids (Angiosan) in patients with psoriasis and psoriatic arthritis. *Journal of International Medical Research* 1990; 18:68–73.

Lau CS, Morley KD, Belch JJF. Effects of fish oil supplementation on non-steroidal anti-inflammatory drug requirement in patients with mild rheumatoid arthritis—a double-blind placebo controlled study. *British Journal of Rheumatology* 1993; 32:982–89.

LaVecchia C, Franceschi S, Decarli A, et al. Dietary vitamin A and the risk of invasive cervical cancer. *International Journal of Cancer* 1984; 34:319–22.

Lawrence R, Sorrell T. Eicasopentaenoic acid in cystic fibrosis; evidence of a pathogenetic role for leukotriene B4. *Lancet* 1993; 342:465–69.

Lee HP, Gourley L, Duffy SW, et al. Dietary effects on breast cancer risk in Singapore. *Lancet* 1991; 337:1197–1200.

Lind L, Lithell H, Pollare T, Ljunghall S. Blood pressure during long-term treatment with magnesium is dependent on magnesium status. *American Journal of Hypertension* 1991; 4:674–79.

Lipkin M, Newmark H. Effect of added dietary calcium on colonic epithelial-cell proliferation in subjects at high risk for familial colonic cancer. *New England Journal of Medicine* 1985; 313:1381–84.

Lippman SM, Meyskens FL. Retinoids for the prevention of cancer. In *Nutrition and Cancer Prevention: investigating the role of micronutrients*, edited by TE Moon, MS Micozzi. Marcel Dekker, 1989, New York and Basel:243–73.

Litovitz TL, Kolm KC, Bailey KM, Schmitz BF. Annual report of poison control centers national data collection system. *American Journal of Emergence Medicine* 1992; 10:452–505.

Lozoff B, Jiminez E, Wolf AW. Long-term developmental outcome of infants with iron deficiency. *New England Journal of Medicine* 1991; 325:687–94.

Matsuoka LY, Wortsman J, Hanifan N, et al. Chronic sunscreen use decreases circulating concentrations of 25-hydroxyvitamin D. *Archives of Dermatology* 1988; 124:1802–04.

Mattingley PC, Mowat AG. Zinc sulphate in rheumatoid arthritis. *Annals of the Rheumatic Diseases* 1982; 41:456–57.

Maurice PDL, Allen BR, Barkley ASJ, et al. The effects of dietary supplementation with fish oil in patients with psoriasis. *British Journal of Dermatology* 1987; 117:599–606.

McKenney JM, Proctor JD, Harris S, Chinchili VM. A comparison of the efficacy and toxic effects of sustained- vs. immediate-release niacin in hypercholesterolemic patients. *Journal of the American Medical Association* 1994; 271:672–77.

Menkes MS, Comstock GW, Vuilleumier JP. Serum beta-carotene, vitamins A and E, selenium, and the risk of lung cancer. *New England Journal of Medicine* 1986; 315:1250–54.

Meydani M. Vitamin E. *Lancet* 1995; 345:170–75.

Meyskens FL Jr, Surwit E, Moon TE, et al. Enhancement of regression of cervical intraepithelial neoplasia II (moderate dysplasia) with topically applied all-trans retinoic acid: a randomized trial. *Journal of the National Cancer Institute* 1994; 86:539–43.

Mikami H, Ogihara T, Tabuchi Y. Blood pressure response to dietary calcium intervention in humans. *American Journal of Hypertension* 1990;3:147S–51S.

Miller J. Allergic arthritis. *Annals of Allergy* 1949:497–501.

Mills JL, Mcpartlin JM, Kirke PN, et al. Homocysteine metabolism in pregnancies complicated by neural-tube defects. *Lancet* 1995; 345:149–51.

Milman N, Scheibel J, Jessen O. Lysine prophylaxis in recurrent herpes simplex labialis. *Lancet* 1978:942.

Milman N, Scheibel J, Jessen O. Lysine prophylaxis in recurrent herpes labialis: a double-blind, controlled crossover study. *Acta Dermatovener* (Stockholm) 1980; 60:85–87.

Montes LF, Diaz ML, Lajous J, Garcia NJ. Folic acid and vitamin B_{12} in vitiligo: a nutritional approach. *Cutis* 1992; 50:39–42.

Morisco C, Trimarco B, Condrelli M. Effect of coenzyme Q10 therapy in patients with congestive heart failure: a long-term multi-center randomized study. *Clinical Investigator* 1993; 71:S134–S136.

Morris MC, Sacks F, Rosner B. Does fish oil lower blood pressure? *Circulation* 1993; 88:523–33.

Nelson RL, Davis FG, Sutter E, et al. Body iron stores and risk of colonic neoplasia. *Journal of the National Cancer Institute* 1994; 86:455–60.

Nielsen GL, Faarvang KL Thomsen BS, et al. The effects of dietary supplementation with n-3 polyunsaturated fatty acids in patients with rheumatoid arthritis: a randomized, double blind trial. *European Journal of Clinical Investigation* 1992; 22:687–91.

Nolan CR, DeGoes J, Alfrey AC. Aluminum and lead absorption from dietary sources in women ingesting calcium citrate. *Southern Medical Journal* 1994; 87(9):894–98.

O'Hara JO, Jolly PN, Nicol CG. The therapeutic efficacy of inositol nicotinate (Hexopal) in intermittent claudication: a controlled trial. *The British Journal of Clinical Practice* 1988; 42:377–83.

O'Keeffe ST, Gavin K, Lavan JN. Iron status and restless legs syndrome in the elderly. *Age and Ageing* 1994; 23:200–203.

Olsen SF, Sorensen JD, Secher NJ, et al. Randomized controlled trial of effect of fish-oil supplementation on pregnancy duration. *Lancet* 1992; 339:1003–07.

Ornish D, Brown SB, Scherwitz LW, et al. Can lifestyle change reverse coronary heart disease? *Lancet* 1990; 336:129–33.

Perticone F, Adinolfi L, Bonaduce D. Efficacy of magnesium sulfate in the treatment of torsade de pointes. *American Heart Journal* 1986;112(4):847–49.

Rasker JJ, Kardaun SH. Lack of beneficial effect of zinc sulphate in rheumatoid arthritis. *Scandinavian Journal of Rheumatology* 1982; 11:168–70.

Rimm EB, Stampfer MJ, Ascherio A, et al. Vitamin E consumption and the risk of coronary heart disease in men. *New England Journal of Medicine* 1993; 328:1450–56.

Riordan AM, Hunter JO, Cowan RE, et al. Treatment of active Crohn's disease by exclusion diet: East Anglian multicentre controlled trial. *Lancet* 1993; 342:1131–34.

Roeback JR, Hla KM, Chambless LE, Fletcher RH. Effects of chromium supplementation on serum high-density lipoprotein cholesterol levels in men taking beta-blockers. *Annals of Internal Medicine* 1991; 115:917–24.

Russell RM, Suter PM. Vitamin requirements of elderly people: an update. *American Journal of Clinical Nutrition* 1993; 58:4–14.

Sahakian V, Rouse D, Sipes S, et al. Vitamin B_6 is effective therapy for nausea and vomiting of pregnancy: a randomized, double-blind placebo-controlled study. *Obstetrics and Gynecology* 1991; 78:33–36.

Salonen JT, Salonen R, Korpela H, et al. Serum copper and the risk of acute myocardial infarction: a prospective population study in men in Eastern Finland. *American Journal of Epidemiology* 1991; 134:268–76.

Seddon JM, Christen WG, Manson JE, et al. The use of vitamin supplementation and the risk of cataract among US male physicians. *American Journal of Public Health* 1994; 84:788–92.

Selhub J, Jacques PF, Wilson PWF, et al. Vitamin status and intake as primary determinants of homocysteinemia in an elderly population. *Journal of the American Medical Association* 270; 22:2693–98.

Semba RD, Miotti PG, Chiphangwi JD, et al. Maternal vitamin A deficiency and mother-to-child transmission of HIV-1. *Lancet* 1994; 343:1593–97.

Senti FR, Pilch SM. Analysis of folate data from the Second Nutritional Health and Nutrition Examination Survey (NHANES) *Journal of Nutrition* 1985; 115:1398–1402.

Sestilli MA. Possible adverse health effects of vitamin C and ascorbic acid. *Seminars in Oncology* 1983; 10(3):299–304.

Shahar E, Folsom AR, Melnick SL, et al. Dietary n-3 polyunsaturated fatty acids and smoking-related chronic obstructive pulmonary disease. *New England Journal of Medicine* 1994; 331:228–33.

Shahar E, Folsom AR, Wu KK, et al. Associations of fish intake and dietary n-3 polyunsaturated fatty acids with a hypocoagulable profile. *Arteriosclerosis and Thrombosis* 1993; 13:1205–12.

Shemesh Z, Attias J, Ornan M, et al. Vitamin B_{12} deficiency in patients with chronic tinnitus and noise-induced hearing loss. *American Journal of Otolaryngology* 1993; 14:94–99.

Simkin PA. Oral zinc sulphate in rheumatoid arthritis. *Lancet* 1976:539–42.

Skobeloff EM, Spivey WH, McNamara RM, Greenspon L. Intravenous magnesium sulfate for the treatment of acute asthma in the emergency department. *Journal of the American Medical Association* 1989; 262:1210–13.

Smith DS, Helzner EC, Nuttall CE. Failure of zinc gluconate in treatment of acute upper respiratory tract infections. *Antimicrobial Agents and Chemotherapy* 1989; 33(5):646–48.

Soyland E, Funk J, Rajka G, et al. Effect of dietary supplementation with very-long-chain n-3 fatty acids in patients with psoriasis. *New England Journal of Medicine* 1993; 328:1812–16.

Stampfer MJ, Hennekens CH, Manson JE, et al. Vitamin E consumption and the risk of coronary disease in women. *New England Journal of Medicine* 1993; 328:1444–49.

Stampfer MJ, Malinow MR, Willett WC, et al. A prospective study of plasma homocysteine and risk of myocardial infarction in US physicians. *Journal of the American Medical Association* 1992; 268:877–81.

Steiner M, Glantz M, Lekos A. Vitamin E and aspirin compared with aspirin alone in patients with transient ischemic attacks. *American Journal of Clinical Nutrition* Dec 1995; 62(6Supp):1381S–1384S.

Stenson WF, Cort D, Rodgers J, et al. Dietary supplementation with fish oil in ulcerative colitis. *Annals of Internal Medicine* 1992; 116:609–14.

Stevens RG, Jones DY, Micozzi MS, Taylor PR. Body iron stores and the risk of cancer. *New England Journal of Medicine* 1988; 319:1047–52.

Suadicani P, Hein HO, Gyntelberg F. Serum selenium concentration and risk of ischaemic heart disease in a prospective cohort study of 3000 males. *Atherosclerosis* 1992; 96:33–42.

Swank RL, Dugan BB. Effect of low saturated fat diet in early and late cases of multiple sclerosis. *Lancet* 1990; 336:37–39.

THPCRG. Trials of hypertension prevention collaborative research group. The effects of nonpharmacologic interventions on blood pressure of persons with high normal levels. Results of the trials of hypertension prevention, phase 1. *Journal of the American Medical Association* 1992; 267:1213–20.

Tsivoni D, Banai S, Schuger C, et al. Treatment of torsades de pointes with magnesium sulfate. *Circulation* 1988; 77(2):392–97.

Ubbink JB, van der Merwe A, Vermaak WJH, Delport R. Hyperhomocysteinemia and the response to vitamin supplementation. *Clinical Investigator* 1993; 71:993–98.

van der Heide JJH, Bilo HJG, Donker JM, et al. Effect of dietary fish oil on renal function and rejection in cyclosporine-treated recipients of renal transplants. *New England Journal of Medicine* 1993; 329:769–73.

Wadleigh RG, Redman RS, Graham ML, et al. Vitamin E in the treatment of chemotherapy-induced mucositis. *American Journal of Medicine* 1992;92:481–84.

Wandzilak TR, D'Andre SD, Davis PA, Williams HE. Effect of high-dose vitamin C on urinary oxalate levels. *Journal of Urology* 1994;151:834–37.

Wargovich MJ. Calcium, vitamin D, and the prevention of gastrointestinal cancer. In *Nutrition and Cancer Prevention: investigating the role of micronutrients*, edited by TE Moon, MS Micozzi. Marcel Dekker, 1989, New York and Basel:291–304.

Whang R, Ryder KW. Frequency of hypomagnesemia and hypermagnesemia: requested vs. routine. *Journal of the American Medical Association* 1990; 263(22):3063–64.

Willis RS, Winn WW, Morris AT, et al. Clinical observations in treatment of nausea and vomiting in pregnancy with vitamins B_1 and B_6. *American Journal of Obstetrics and Gynecology* 1942; 44:265–71.

Witteman, JCM, Grobbee DE, Derkx FHM, et al. Reduction of blood pressure with oral magnesium supplementation in women with mild to moderate hypertension. *American Journal of Clinical Nutrition* 1994; 60:129–35.

Woods KL, Fletcher S, Roffe C, Haider Y. Intravenous magnesium sulfate in suspected acute myocardial infarction: results of the second Leicester Intravenous Magnesium Intervention Trial (LIMIT-2). *Lancet* 1992; 339:1553–58.

Woods KL, Fletcher S. Long-term outcome after intravenous magnesium sulphate in suspected acute myocardial infarction: the second Leicester Intravenous Magnesium Intervention Trial (Limit-2). *Lancet* 1994; 343:816–19.

Wouters MGAJ, Boers GHJ, Blom HJ, et al. Hyperhomocysteinemia: a risk factor in women with unexplained recurrent early pregnancy loss. *Fertility and Sterility* 1993; 60:820–25.

Zarembo JE, Godfrey JC, Godfrey NJ. Zinc (II) in saliva: determination of concentrations produced by different formulations of zinc gluconate lozenges containing common excipients. *Journal of Pharmaceutical Sciences* 1992; 81(2):128–30.

Zeller M. Rheumatoid arthritis—food allergy as a factor. *Annals of Allergy* 1949:200–205.

Exercise

Albanes D, Blair A, Taylor PR. Physical activity and risk of cancer in the NHANES I population. *American Journal of Public Health* 1989; 79:744–50.

Berlin JA, Colditz G. A meta-analysis of physical activity in the prevention of coronary heart disease. *American Journal of Epidemiology* 1990; 132:612–28.

Bernstein L, Henderson BE, Hanisch R, et al. Physical exercise and reduced risk of breast cancer in young women. *Journal of the National Cancer Institute* 1994; 86(18):1403–08.

Brubaker L, Kotarinos R. Kegel or cut? Variations on his theme. *Journal of Reproductive Medicine* 1993; 38(9):672–78.

Chow R, Harrison JE, Notarius C. Effect of two randomized exercise programmes on bone mass of healthy postmenopausal women. *British Medical Journal* 1987; 295:1441–44.

Claes H, Baert L. Pelvic floor exercise versus surgery in the treatment of impotence. *British Journal of Urology* 1993; 71:52–57.

Curfman GD. The health benefits of exercise: a critical reappraisal. *New England Journal of Medicine* 1993; 22:468–77.

Elia G, Bergman A. Pelvic muscle exercises: when do they work? *Obstetrics and Gynecology* 1993; 81(2):283–86.

Fiatarone MA, Marks EC, Ryan ND, et al. High-intensity strength training in nonagenarians: effects on skeletal muscle. *Journal of the American Medical Association* 1990; 263:3029–34.

Fiatarone MA, O'Neill EF, Ryan ND, et al. Exercise training and nutritional supplementation for physical frailty in very elderly people. *New England Journal of Medicine* 1994; 330:1769–75.

Garcia-Palmieri MR, Costas R Jr, Cruz-Vidal M, Sorlie PD, Havlik RJ. Increased physical activity: a protective factor against heart attacks in Puerto Rico. *American Journal of Cardiology* 1982; 50:749–55.

Griest J, Klein M, Eischens R, Faris J. Antidepressant running: running as treatment for non-psychotic depression. *Behavioral Medicine* 1978; 5:19–24.

Hambrecht R, Niebauer J, Marburger C, et al. Various intensities of leisure time physical activity in patients with coronary artery disease: effects on cardiorespiratory fitness and progression of coronary atherosclerotic lesions. *Journal of the American College of Cardiology* 1993; 22:468–77.

Helmrich SP, Ragland DR, Leung RW, Paffenberger RS. Physical activity and reduced occurrence of non-insulin-dependent diabetes mellitus. *New England Journal of Medicine* 1991; 325:147–52.

Kiely DK, Wolf PA, Cupples LA, et al. Physical activity and stroke: the Framingham study. *American Journal of Epidemiology* 1994; 140(7):608–20.

Klarskov P, Belving D, Bischoff N et al. Pelvic floor exercise versus surgery for female urinary stress incontinence. *Urologia Internationalis* 1986;41:129–32.

Klein MH, Griest JH, Gurman AS, et al. A comparative outcome study of group psychotherapy vs. exercise treatments for depression. *International Journal of Mental Health* 1985; 13(3-4):148–77.

Lakka TA, Venalainen JM, Rauramaa R, et al. Relation of leisure-time physical activity and cardiorespiratory fitness to the risk of acute myocardial infarction in men. *New England Journal of Medicine* 1994; 330:1549–54.

Leon AS, Connett J, Jacobs DR Jr, Rauramaa R. Leisure-time physical activity levels and risk of coronary heart disease and death: the Multiple Risk Factor Intervention Trial. *Journal of the American Medical Association* 1987; 258:2388–95.

Manson JE, Nathan DM, Krolewski AS, et al. A prospective study of exercise and incidence of diabetes among US male physicians. *Journal of the American Medical Association* 1992; 268:63–67.

McCann IL, Holmes DS. Influence of aerobic exercise on depression. *Journal of Personality and Social Psychology* 1984; 46(5):1142–47.

McMurdo MET, Rennie L. A controlled trial of exercise by residents of old people's homes. *Age and Ageing* 1993; 22:11–15.

Mittleman MA, Maclure M, Tofler GH, et al. Triggering of acute myocardial infarction by heavy physical exertion; protection against triggering by regular exertion. *New England Journal of Medicine* 1993; 329:1677–83.

Paffenbarger RS Jr, Wing AL, Hsieh CC. Physical activity, all-cause mortality, and longevity of college alumni. *New England Journal of Medicine* 1986; 314:605–13.

Ross CE and Hayes D. Exercise and psychological well-being in the community. *American Journal of Epidemiology* 1988; 127:762–71.

Salonen JT, Slater JS, Tuomilehto J, Rauramaa R. Leisure time and occupational physical activity: risk of death from ischemic heart disease. *American Journal of Epidemiology* 1988; 127:87–94.

Sandvik L, Erikssen J, Thaulow E, et al. Physical fitness as a predictor of mortality among healthy, middle-aged Norwegian men. *New England Journal of Medicine* 1993; 328:533–37.

Schneider MS, King LR, Surwit RS. Kegel exercises and childhood incontinence: a new role for an old treatment. *Journal of Pediatrics* 1994; 124:91–92.

Slattery ML, Jacobs DR, Nichaman MZ. Leisure time physical activity and coronary heart disease death. *Circulation* 1989; 79:304–11.

Stanley, Edward (Earl of Derby). The Conduct of Life. Address at Liverpool College, December 20, 1873.

Willich SN, Lewis M, Lowel H, et al. Physical exertion as a trigger of acute myocardial infarction. *New England Journal of Medicine* 1993; 329:1684–90.

Herbs

Amure BO. Clinical study of Duogastrone in the treatment of duodenal ulcers. *Gut* 1970;11:171–75.

Arena JM. Plants that poison. *Emergency Medicine* 1989; Jun 15:20–64.

Auer W, Eiber A, Hertkorn E, et al. Hypertension and hyperlipidaemia: garlic helps in mild cases. *British Journal of Clinical Practice* 1990; (Supplement 69):3–6.

Avorn J, Monane M, Gurwitz JH. Reduction of bacteriuria and pyuria after ingestion of cranberry juice. *Journal of the American Medical Association* 1994; 271(10):751–54.

Awang DVC. Herbal medicine: feverfew. *Canadian Pharmaceutical Journal* 1989; 122:266–70.

Bannister B, Ginsburg R, Shneerson J. Cardiac arrest due to liquorice-induced hypokalaemia. *British Medical Journal* 1977; 2:738–39.

Belch JJF, Ansell D, Madhok R, et al. Effects of altering dietary essential fatty acids on requirements for non-steroidal anti-inflammatory drugs in patients with rheumatoid arthritis. *Annals of Rheumatic Disease* 1988; 47:96–104.

Bernstein JE, Korman NJ, Bickers DR, et al. Topical capsaicin treatment of chronic postherpetic neuralgia. *Journal of the American Academy of Dermatology* 1989; 21:265–70.

Bone ME, Wilkinson DJ, Young JR, et al. Ginger root: a new antiemetic. The effect of ginger root on postoperative nausea and vomiting after major gynecological surgery. *Anaesthesia* 1990; 45:669–71.

Bordia A, Bansal HC, Arora SK, Singh SV. Effect of the essential oils of garlic and onion on alimentary hyperlipemia. *Atherosclerosis* 1975; 21:15–19.

Bordia A. Effect of garlic on blood lipids in patients with coronary heart disease. *American Journal of Clinical Nutrition* 1981; 34:2100–03.

Bordia A. Effect of garlic on human platelet aggregation in vitro. *Atherosclerosis* 1978; 30:355–60.

Bower B. Herbal medicine: Rx for chimps? *Science News* 1986; Jan 18; 129:138.

Brzeski M, Madhok R, Capell HA. Evening primrose oil in patients with rheumatoid arthritis and side effects of non-steroidal anti-inflammatory drugs. *British Journal of Rheumatology* 1991; 30:370–72.

Bultitude MI. Capsaicin in treatment of loin pain/haematuria syndrome. *Lancet* 1995; 345:921–22.

Champault G, Patel JC, Bonnard AM. A double-blind trial of an extract of the plant Serenoa repens in benign prostatic hyperplasia. *British Journal of Clinical Pharmacology* 1984; 18:461–62.

Cliff JM and Milton-Thomson GJ. A double-blind trial of carbenoxolone sodium capsules in the treatment of duodenal ulcer. *Gut* 1970; 11:167–70.

Conn EE. Cyanogenetic glycosides. In *Toxicants Occurring Naturally in Foods*, Committee on Food Protection, Food and Nutrition Board, National Resource Council, National Academy of Sciences, Washington DC 1973:304–07.

CSG. Capsaicin Study Group. Treatment of painful diabetic neuropathy with topical capsaicin. *Archives of Internal Medicine* 1991; 151:2225–29.

Doll R, Hill ID, Hutton C, Underwood DJ. Clinical trial of a triterpenoid liquorice compound in gastric and duodenal ulcer. *Lancet* 1962:793–96.

Dumont E, Petit E, Tarrade T, Nouvelot A. UV-C irradiation-induced peroxidative degradation of microsomal fatty acids and proteins: protection by an extract of Ginkgo biloba (EGb 761). *Free Radical Biology and Medicine* 1992; 13:197–203.

Epstein MT, Espiner EA, Donald RA, Hughes H. Effect of eating liquorice on the renin-angiotensin aldosterone axis in normal subjects. *British Medical Journal* 1977; 1:488–90.

Ernst E. St. Johnswort, an antidepressant? A systematic, criteria-based review. *Phytomedicine* 1995; 2(1):67–71.

Fackelmann KA. Food, drug, or poison? Cultivating a taste for 'toxic' plants. *Science News* 1993; 143:312–14.

Farese RV, Biglieri EG, Shackleton CHL, et al. Licorice-induced hypermineralocorticoidism. *New England Journal of Medicine* 1991; 325(17):1223–27.

Ferenci P, Dragosics B, Dittrich H, et al. Randomized controlled trial of silymarin treatment in patients with cirrhosis of the liver. *Journal of Hepatology* 1989; 9:105–113.

Fischer-Rasmussen W, Kjaer SK, Dahl C, Asping U. Ginger treatment of hyperemesis gravidarum. *European Journal of Obstetrics & Gynecology and Reproductive Biology* 1990; 38:19–24.

Folkenberg J. FDA Consumer. Oct 1988:16–17.

Foster S, Duke JA. *Eastern/Central medicinal plants* (Peterson field guides). Houghton Mifflin Co, 1990, Boston:vii.

Gately CA, Miers M, Mansel RE, Hughes LE. Drug treatments for mastalgia: 17 years experience in the Cardiff mastalgia clinic. *Journal of the Royal Society of Medicine* 1992; 85:12–15.

Gordon DW, Rosenthal G, Hart J, et al. Chaparral ingestion: the broadening spectrum of liver injury caused by herbal medications. *Journal of the American Medical Association* 1995; 273(6):489–90.

Greenspan EM. Ginseng and vaginal bleeding. *Journal of the American Medical Association* 1983; 249:2018.

Grontved A, Brask T, Kambskard J, Hentzer E. Ginger root against seasickness: a controlled trial on the open sea. *Acta Otolaryngology* 1988; 105:45–49.

Grontved A, Hentzer E. Vertigo-reducing effect of ginger root: a controlled clinical study. *Journal of Oto-Rhino-Laryngology and its Related Specialties* 1986; 48:282–86.

Hofferberth B. The efficacy of EGb 761 in patients with senile dementia of the Alzheimer type: a double-blind, placebo-controlled study on different levels of investigation. *Human Psychopharmacology* 1994; 9:215–22.

Hopkins MP, Androff L, Bennighoff AS. Ginseng face cream and unexplained vaginal bleeding. *American Journal of Obstetrics and Gynecology* 1988; 159:1121–22.

Huxtable RJ. Herbal teas and toxins: novel aspects of pyrrolizidine poisoning in the United States.. *Perspectives in Biology and Medicine*; 24(1):1–14.

Huxtable RJ. The harmful potential of herbal and other plant products. *Drug Safety* 1990; 5 (suppl 1):126–36.

Jacobsen TD, Krenzelok EP. Botanical villains? Common plant exposures, Part 1. *Family Practice Recertification* 1992; 14 (8):74–86.

Jaffé WG. Hemagglutinins. In *Toxic Constituents of Plant Foodstuffs* by IE Liener, Academic Press, 1969, New York and London:78–82.

Jain AK, Vargas R, et al. Can garlic reduce levels of serum lipids? A controlled clinical study. *American Journal of Medicine* 1993; 94:632–35.

Jiang J-B, Li G-Q, Guo X-B, et al. Antimalarial activity of mefloquine and quinhaosu. *Lancet* 1982:285–88.

Johnson ES, Kadam NP, Hylands DM, Hylands PJ. Efficacy of feverfew as prophylactic treatment of migraine. *British Medical Journal* 1985; 291:569–73.

Johnson MG and Vaughn RH. Death of Salmonella typhimurium and Escherichia coli in the presence of freshly reconstituted dehydrated garlic and onion. *Applied Microbiology* 1969; 17(6):903–05.

Kassir ZA. Endoscopic controlled trial of four drug regimens in the treatment of chronic duodenal ulcers. *Irish Medical Journal* 1985; 78:153–56.

Katz M, Saibil F. Herbal hepatitis:subacute hepatic necrosis secondary to chaparral leaf. *Journal of Clinical Gastroenterology* 1990; 12:203–06.

Kiesewetter H, Jung EM, Mrowietz C, et al. Effect of garlic on platelet aggregation in patients with increased risk of juvenile ischemic attack. *European Journal of Clinical Pharmacology* 1993; 45:333–36.

Kleijnen J, Knipschild P. Ginkgo biloba for cerebral insufficiency. *British Journal of Clinical Pharmacology* 1992; 34:352–58.

Kleijnen J, Knipschild P. Ginkgo biloba. *Lancet* 1992; 340:1136–39.

Kong X-T, Fang HT, Jiang GQ, et al. Treatment of acute bronchiolitis with Chinese herbs. *Archives of Disease in Childhood* 1993; 68:468–71.

Larrey D, Vial T, Pauwels A, et al. Hepatitis after germander administration: another instance of herbal medicine hepatotoxicity. *Annals of Internal Medicine* 1992; 117(2)129–32.

Leathwood PD, Chauffard F, Herck E, Munoz-Box R. Aqueous extract of valerian root improves sleep quality in man. *Pharmacology Biochemistry and Behavior* 1982; 17:65–71.

Leventhal LJ, Boyce EG, and Zurier RB. Treatment of rheumatoid arthritis with gammalinolenic acid. *Annals of Internal Medicine* 1993;119(9):867–73.

Li G-Q, Arnold K, Guo X-B. Randomized comparative study of mefloquine, quinghaosu, and pyrimethamine-sulfadoxine in patients with falciparum malaria. *Lancet* 1984:1360–61.

Lindahl O, Lindwall L. Double blind study of a valerian preparation. *Pharmacology, Biochemistry and Behavior* 1989; 32:1065–66.

Lovell CR, Burton JL, Horrobin DF. Treatment of atopic eczema with evening primrose oil. *Lancet* 1981:278.

Mayeux PR, Agrawal KC, Tou J-SH, et al. The pharmacological effects of allicin, a constituent of garlic oil. *Agents and Actions* 1988; 25(1–2):182–90.

McCaleb RS. Food ingredient safety evaluation. *Food and Drug Law Journal* 1992; 47 (6):657–63.

McCarthy GM and McCarty DJ. Effect of topical capsaicin in the therapy of painful osteoarthritis of the hands. *Journal of Rheumatology* 1992; 19:604–07.

McCarty DJ, Csuka M, McCarthy G, Trotter D. Treatment of pain due to fibromyalgia with topical capsaicin: a pilot study. *Seminars in Arthritis and Rheumatism* 1994; 23(6), Suppl 3:41–47.

Melchart D, Linde K, Worku F, et al. Immunomodulation with Echinacea—a systematic review of controlled clinical trials. *Phytomedicine* 1994; 1:245–54.

Morgan AG, McAdam WAF, Pacsoo C, Darborough A. Comparison between cimetidine and Caved-S in the treatment of gastric ulceration, and subsequent maintenance therapy. *Gut* 1982; 23:545–51.

Mowrey DB. Motion sickness, ginger,and psychophysics. *Lancet* 1982:655–57.

Murphy JJ, Heptinsall S, Mitchell JRA. Randomized double-blind placebo-controlled trial of feverfew in migraine prevention. *Lancet* 1988:189–92.

Nishino H, Iwashima A, Itakura Y, et al. Antitumor-promoting activity of garlic extracts. *Oncology* 1989; 46:277–80.

Ofek I, Goldhar J, Zafriri D, et al. Anti-escherichia coli adhesion activity of cranberry and blueberry juices. *New England Journal of Medicine* 1991; 324(22):1599.

Phelps S, Harris WS. Garlic supplementation and lipoprotein oxidation susceptibility. *Lipids* 1993; 28(5) 475–77.

Punnonen R, Lukola A. Oestrogen-like effect of ginseng. *British Medical Journal* 1980; 281:1110.

Rees WDW, Rhodes J, Wright JE, et al. Effect of deglycyrrhizinated liquorice on gastric mucosal damage by aspirin. *Scandinavian Journal of Gastroenterology* 1979; 14:605.

Salmi HA, Sarna S. Effect of silymarin on chemical, functional, and morphological alterations of the liver. *Scandinavian Journal of Gastroenterology* 1982; 17:517–20.

Schalin-Karrila M, Mattila L, Jansen CT, Uotila P. Evening primrose oil in the treatment of atopic eczema: effect on clinical status, plasma phospholipid fatty acids and circulating blood prostaglandins. *British Journal of Dermatology* 1987; 117:11–19.

Sheehan MP, Atherton DJ. A controlled trial of traditional Chinese medicine plants in widespread, non-exudative atopic eczema. *British Journal of Dermatology* 1992; 126:179–84.

Sheehan MP, Rustin MHA, Atherton DJ. Efficacy of traditional Chinese herbal treatment in adult atopic dermatitis. *Lancet* 1992; 340:13–17.

Sikora R, Sohn M, Deutz F-J, et al. Ginkgo biloba extract in the therapy of erectile dysfunction. *Journal of Urology* 1989; 141:188A (abstract).

Sobota AE. Inhibition of bacterial adherence by cranberry juice: potential use for the treatment of urinary tract infections. *Journal of Urology* 1984; 131:1013–16.

Stewart JJ, Wood MJ, Wood, CD. Mims ME. Effects of ginger on motion sickness susceptibility and gastric function. *Pharmacology* 1991; 42:111–20.

Sy ND, Hoan DB, Dung NP, et al. Treatment of malaria in Vietnam with oral artemisinin. *American Journal of Tropical Medicine and Hygiene* 1993; 48(3):398–402.

Tewari SN and Wilson AK. Deglycyrrhizinated liquorice in duodenal ulcer. *Practitioner* 1973; 210:820–23.

Tuchweber B, Sieck R, Trost W. Prevention by silybin of phalloidin-induced acute hepatotoxicity. *Toxicology and Applied Pharmacology* 1979; 51:265–75.

Turpie AGG, Runcie J,Thompson TJ. Clinical trial of deglycyrrhizinized liquorice in gastric ulcer. *Gut* 1969; 10:299–302.

Vorberg G, Scneider B. Therapy with garlic: results of a placebo-controlled, double-blind study. *British Journal of Clinical Practice* 1990; (Supplement 69):7–11.

Wargovich MJ. Diallyl sulfide, a flavor component of garlic (allium sativum) inhibits dimethylhydrazine-induced colon cancer. *Carcinogenesis* 1987; 8(3):487–89.

Warshafsky S, Kamer RS, Sivak SL. Effect of garlic on total serum cholesterol: a meta-analysis. *Annals of Internal Medicine* 1993; 119:599–605.

Watson CPN, Evan RJ. The postmastectomy pain syndrome and topical capsaicin: a randomized trial. *Pain* 1992; 51:372–79.

Watson CPN, Evans RJ, Watt VR. Post-herpetic neuralgia and topical capsaicin. *Pain* 1988; 33:333–40.

Weiss, RF. *Herbal Medicine*. Beaconsfield Publishers, 1991, Beaconsfield, England:333. (Original German edition first published in 1960.)

Woolf GM, Petrovic LM, Rojter SE, et al. Acute hepatitis associated with the Chinese herbal product Jin Bu Huan. *Annals of Internal Medicine* 1994; 121:729–35.

Wright S, Burton JL. Oral evening-primrose-seed oil improves atopic eczema. *Lancet* 1982:1120–22.

You W-C, Blot WJ, Chang Y-S, et al. Allium vegetables and reduced risk of stomach cancer. *Journal of the National Cancer Institute* 1989; 81:162–64.

Yun,T-K, Choi SY. Preventive effect of ginseng intake against various human cancers: a case-control study on 1987 pairs. *Cancer Epidemiology, Biomarkers, and Prevention* 1995; 4(4):401–08.

Zatuchni GI, Colombi DJ. Bromelain therapy for the prevention of episiotomy pain. *Obstetrics and Gynecology* 1967; 29(2):275–78.

Homeopathy

Benveniste J. Dr Jacques Benveniste replies. *Nature* 1988; 324:291.

Boyd H. Homeopathy in general medical practice. *World Health Forum* (publication of the World Health Organization) 1983; 4(2):102–05.

Brigo B, Serpelloni G. Homeopathic treatment of migraines: a randomized double-blind controlled study of sixty cases. *The Berlin Journal on Research in Homeopathy* 1991; 1(2):98–105.

Coulter H. *Homeopathic Science and Modern Medicine: the physics of healing with microdoses*. North Atlantic Books, 1980, Berkeley CA:19, 24.

Davenas E, Beauvais F, Amara J, et al. Human basophil degranulation triggered by very dilute antiserum against IgE. *Nature* 1988; 333:816–18.

Day CEI. Control of stillbirths in pigs using homeopathy. *Veterinary Record* 1984; 114:216.

de Lange de Klerk ESM, Blommers J, Kuik DJ, et al. Effect of homoeopathic medicines on daily burden of symptoms in children with recurrent upper respiratory tract infections. *British Medical Journal* 1994; 309:1329–32.

FDA. Riding the coattails of homeopathy's revival. *FDA Consumer* 1985:30–34.

Ferley P, Zmirou D, D'Adhemar D, Balducci F. A controlled evaluation of a homeopathic preparation in the treatment of influenza-like syndromes. *British Journal of Clinical Pharmacology* 1989; 27:329–35.

Fisher P, Greenwood A, Huskisson EC, et al. Effect of homeopathic treatment on fibrositis (primary fibromyalgia). *British Medical Journal* 1989; 299:365–66.

Gipson RG, Gipson SLM, MacNeill AD, Buchanan WW. Homeopathic therapy in rheumatoid arthritis: evaluation by double-blind clinical therapeutic trial. *British Journal of Clinical Pharmacology* 1980; 9:453–59.

Hahnemann S, "Was sind Giften, was sind Arzneien?" (What are poisons, what are medicines?) *Journal der practischen Heilkunde* XXIV 1806; st.III:40–57. Quoted in Coulter 1980:46.

Jacobs J, Jiminez M, Gloyd SS, et al. Treatment of acute childhood diarrhea with homeopathic medicine: a randomized clinical trial in Nicaragua. *Pediatrics* 1994; 93:719–25.

Jacobs, J. Homeopathy. In *Fundamentals of Complementary and Alternative Medicine*, edited by MS Micozzi. Churchill-Livingstone, 1996, New York.

Kleijnen J, Knipschild P, ter Riet G. Clinical trials of homeopathy. *British Medical Journal* 1992; 302:316–23.

Maddox J, Randi J, Stewart WW. "High-dilution" experiments a delusion. *Nature* 1988; 324:287–90.

Reilly D, Taylor MA, Beattie NGM. Is evidence for homoeopathy reproducible? *Lancet* 1994; 344:1601–06.

Reilly DT, McSharry C, Taylor MA, Aitchison T. Is homeopathy a placebo response? Controlled trial of homeopathic potencies, with pollen in hayfever as a model. *Lancet* 1986:881–86.

Starr P. *The social transformation of American medicine.* Basic Books, Inc/Harper, 1982, New York:98.

Stedman's Medical Dictionary, Williams and Wilkins, 1972, Baltimore MD:583.

Vithoulkas G. Homeopathy today. *World Health Forum* 1983; 4:99–101.

Vithoulkas G. *The Science of Homepathy.* Grove Press, 1980, New York.

Hypnosis and imagery

Andersen MS. Hypnotizability as a factor in the hypnotic treatment of obesity. *International Journal of Clinical and Experimental Hypnosis* 1985; 33:150–59.

Barabasz M, Spiegel D. Hypnotizability and weight loss in obese subjects. *International Journal of Eating Disorders* 1989; 8(3):335–41.

Cochrane G, Friesen J. Hypnotherapy in weight loss treatment. *Journal of Consulting and Clinical Psychology* 1986; 54:489–92.

Day GH. The subjective effects of general irradiation. *British Journal of Physical Medicine* 1955; 18:15.

Erickson MH, Hershman S, Secter II. *The Practical Application of Medical and Dental Hypnosis.* Seminars on Hypnosis Publishing Company, 1981, Chicago:4–10.

Ewer TC, Stewart DE. Improvement in bronchial hyper-responsiveness in patients with moderate asthma after treatment with a hypnotic technique: a randomized controlled trial. *British Medical Journal* 1986; 293:1129–32.

Feher SDK, Berger LR, Johnson JD, Wilde JB. Increasing breast milk production for premature infants with a relaxation/imagery audiotape. *Pediatrics* 1989; 83(1):57–60.

Fuchs K, Paldi E, Abramovici H, Peretz BA. Treatment of hyperemesis gravidarum by hypnosis. *International Journal of Clinical and Experimental Hypnosis* 1980; 28:313–23.

Haanen HCM, Hoenderdos HTW, van Romunde LKJ, et al. Controlled trial of hypnotherapy in the treatment of refractory fibromyalgia. *Journal of Rheumatology* 1991; 18(1):72–75.

Harvey RF, Gunary RM, Hinton RA, Barry RE. Individual and group hypnotherapy in treatment of refractory irritable bowel syndrome. *Lancet* 1989:424–25.

Hilgard ER. *Hypnotic Susceptibility.* Harcourt, Brace, and World, 1965, New York.

Holroyd J. Hypnosis treatment for smoking: an evaluative review. *International Journal of Clinical and Experimental Hypnosis* 1980; (4):341–57.

Maher-Loughnan GP, Macdonald N, Mason AA, Fry L. Controlled trial of hypnosis in the symptomatic treatment of asthma. *British Medical Journal* 1962; 2:371–76.

Mason AA. A case of ichthyosiform erythrodermia of Brocq treated by hypnosis. *British Medical Journal* 1952; 2:422–23.

Morrow GR, Morrell C. Behavioral treatment for the anticipatory nausea and vomiting induced by cancer chemotherapy. *New England Journal of Medicine* 1982; 307:1476–80.

Orlick T and Partington J. Mental links to excellence. *Sport Psychology* 1988; 2:105–30.

Redd WH, Andresen GV, Minigawa RY. Hypnotic control of anticipatory emesis in patients receiving cancer chemotherapy. *Journal of Consulting and Clinical Psychology* 1982; 50(1):14-19.

Redd WH, Rosenberger PH, Hendler CS. Controlling chemotherapy side effects. *American Journal of Clinical Hypnosis* 1982–1983; 25(2–3);161–72.

RRC. Report to Research Committee of the British Tuberculosis Association: Hypnosis for asthma: a controlled trial. *British Medical Journal* 1968; 4:71–76.

Shiekh AA, ed. *Imagery: current theory, research, and application.* John Wiley and Sons, 1983, New York.

Spiegel D, Bloom JR. Group therapy and hypnosis reduce metastatic breast carcinoma pain. *Psychosomatic Medicine* 1982; 45:333–39.

Syrjala KL, Cummings C, Donaldson GW. Hypnosis or cognitive behavioral training for the reduction of pain and nausea during cancer treatment: a controlled clinical trial. *Pain* 1992:137–46.

Torem MS. Hypnosis:lingering myths and established facts. *Psychiatric Medicine* 1992; 10(4):1–11.

Whorwell PJ, Prior A, Colgan SM. Hypnotherapy in severe irritable bowel syndrome: further experience. *Gut* 1987; 28:423–25.

Whorwell PJ, Prior A, Faragher EB. Controlled trial of hypnotherapy in the treatment of severe refractory irritable-bowel syndrome. *Lancet* 1984:1232–34.

Whorwell PJ. Use of hypnotherapy in gastrointestinal disease. *British Journal of Hospital Medicine* 1991; 45:27–29.

Zeltzer L, LeBaron S. Hypnosis and non-hypnotic techniques for reduction of pain and anxiety in children and adolescents with cancer. *Behavioral Pediatrics* 1982; 101(6):1032–35.

Massage and bodywork

Bauer WC, Dracup KA. Physiological effects of back massage in patients with acute myocardial infarction. *Focus on Critical Care* 1987; 14(6):42–46.

Benor DJ. Survey of spiritual healing research. *Complementary Medical Research* 1990; 4(30):9–33.

Brennan B, Demmerle A, Patterson M, et al. Manual healing methods. In *Alternative Medicine: Expanding Medical Horizons: a report to the National Institutes of Health on Alternative Medicine Systems and Practices in the United States* 1994:137. Available from the Office of Alternative Medicine, National Institutes of Health, 6120 Executive Blvd #450, Rockville MD 20892-9904.

Cottingham JT, Porges SW, Richmond K. Shifts in pelvic inclination angle and parasympathetic tone produced by rolfing soft tissue manipulation. *Physical Therapy* 1988; 68(9):1364–70.

Danneskiold-Samsoe B, Christiansen E, Andersen RB. Myofascial pain and the role of myoglobin. *Scandinavian Journal of Rheumatology* 1986; 15:175–78.

de Bruijn R. Deep transverse friction: its analgesic effect. *International Journal of Sports Medicine* 1984; 5(Suppl):35–36.

Dyson R (1978). Bed Sores—the injuries hospital staff inflict on patients. *Nursing Mirror* 1978; 146(24):30–32.

Ernst E, Matrai A, Magyarosy I, et al. Massages cause changes in blood fluidity. *Physiotherapy* 1987; 73(1):43–45.

Ferrell-Torry AT, Glick OJ. The use of therapeutic massage as a nursing intervention to modify anxiety and the perception of cancer pain. *Cancer Nursing* 1993; 16(2):93–101.

Field T, Morrow C, Valdeon C, et al. Massage reduces anxiety in child and adolescent psychiatric patients. *Journal of the American Academy of Child and Adolescent Psychiatry* 1992; 31(1):125–31.

223

Field TM, Schanberg SM, Scafidi F, et al. Tactile/kinesthetic stimulation effects on preterm neonates. *Pediatrics* 1986; 77(5):654–58.

Fraser J, Kerr JR. Psychophysiological effects of back massage on elderly institutionalized patients. *Journal of Advanced Nursing* 1993; 18:238–45.

Grad B. Some biological effects of the "laying on of hands": a review of experiments with animals and plants. *Journal of the American Society for Psychical Research* 1965; 59:95–127.

Heidt P. Effect of therapeutic touch on anxiety level of hospitalized patients. *Nursing Research* 1981; 30 (1):32–37.

Hill CF. Is massage beneficial to critically ill patients in intensive care units? A critical review. *Intensive and Critical Care Nursing* 1993; 9:116–21.

Joachim G. The effects of two stress management techniques on feelings of wellbeing in patients with inflammatory bowel disease. *Nursing Papers* 1983; 15(5):18.

Keller E, Bzdek VM. Effects of therapeutic touch on tension headache pain. *Nursing Research* 1986; 35(2):101–06.

Kramer NA. Comparison of therapeutic touch and casual touch in stress reduction of hospitalized children. *Pediatric Nursing* 1990; 16(5):483–85.

Krieger D. *Therapeutic Touch: How to use your hands to help or heal.* Prentice Hall, 1979, Englewood Cliffs NJ.

Kurz W, Wittlinger G, Litmanovitch YI, et al. Effect of manual lymph drainage massage on urinary excretion of neurohormones and minerals in chronic lymphedema. *Angiology* 1978; 29:764–72.

Li ZM. 235 cases of frozen shoulder treated by manipulation and massage. *Journal of Traditional Chinese Medicine* 1984; 4:213–15.

Meehan TC. Therapeutic touch and postoperative pain:a Rogerian research study. *Nursing Science Quarterly* 1993 (Summer); 6(2):69–78.

Melzack R, Bentley KC. Relief of dental pain by ice massage of either hand or the contralateral arm. *Journal of the Canadian Dental Association* 1983; 4:257–60.

Melzack R, Guite S, Gonshor A. Relief of dental pain by ice massage of the hand. *Canadian Medical Association Journal* 1980; 122;189–91.

Melzack R, Jeans ME, Stratford JG, Monks RC. Ice massage and transcutaneous electrical stimulation: comparison of treatment for low-back pain. *Pain* 1980; 9:209–17.

Nordschow M, Bierman W. Influence of manual massage on muscle relaxation. *Physical Therapy* 1962; 42:653–57.

Olson B. Effects of massage for prevention of pressure ulcers. *Decubitus* 1989; 2(4):32–37.

Perry J, Jones MH, Thomas L. Functional evaluation of rolfing in cerebral palsy. *Developental Medicine & Child Neurology* 1981; 23:717–29.

Pham QT, Peslin R, Puchelle E, et al. Respiratory function and the rheological status of bronchial secretions collected by spontaneous expectoration and after physiotherapy. *Bulletin d Physio-pathologie Respiratoire* 1973; 9:292–311.

Quinn JF. Therapeutic touch as energy exchange: testing the theory. *Advances in Nursing Science* 1984; 6:42–49.

Rausch PB. Effects of tactile and kinesthetic stimulation on premature infants. *Journal of Obstetric, Gynecologic and Neonatal Nursing* 1981; 10:34–37.

Ruth S, Kegerreis S. Facilitating cervical flexion using a Feldenkrais method: awareness through movement. *Journal of Orthopedic and Sports Physical Therapy* 1992; 16(1):25–29.

Weinberg RS, Hunt VV. Effects of structural integration on state trait anxiety. *Journal of Clinical Psychology* 1979; 35:319–22.

Wheeden A, Scafidi FA, Field T, et al. Massage effects on cocaine-exposed preterm neonates. *Developmental and Behavioral Pediatrics* 1993; 14(5):318–22.

White JL, LaBarba RC. The effects of tactile and kinesthetic stimulation on neonatal development in the premature infant. *Developmental Psychobiology* 1976; 9:569–77.

Wirth DP. The effect of non-contact therapeutic touch on the healing rate of full thickness dermal wounds. *Subtle Energies* 1990; 1(1):1–20.

Witt PL, MacKinnon J. Trager psychosocial integration: a method to improve chest mobility of patients with chronic lung disease. *Physical Therapy* 1986; 66(2):214–17.

Yates J. *A Physicians Guide to Therapeutic Massage: its physiological effects and their application to treatment.* Massage Therapists Association of British Columbia, 1990, Vancouver BC, Canada.

Zanolla R, Monzeglio C, Balzarini A, Martino G. Evaluation of the results of three different methods of postmastectomy lymphedema treatment. *Journal of Surgical Oncology* 1984; 26:210–13.

The mind/body connection

Albright GL, Fischer AA. Effects of warming imagery aimed at trigger-point sites on tissue compliance, skin temperature, and pain sensitivity in biofeedback-trained patients with chronic pain: a preliminary study. *Perceptual and Motor Skills* 1990; 71:1163–70.

Allen K, Blascovich J. Effects of music on cardiovascular reactivity among surgeon. *Journal of the American Medical Association* 1994; 272:882–84.

Berk LS, Tan SA, Fry WF, et al. Neuroendocrine and stress hormone changes during mirthful laughter. *American Journal of the Medical Sciences* 1989; 298(6):390–96.

Berkman LF, Syme SL. Social networks, host resistance and mortality: a nine year follow-up study of Alameda county residents. *American Journal of Epidemiology* 1979; 109(2):186–204.

Cannon WB. Voodoo Death. *American Anthropologist* 1942; 44(2):169–81.

Case RB, Moss AJ, Case N, et al. Living alone after myocardial infarction. *Journal of the American Medical Association* 1992; 267:515–19.

Cheren S. *Psychosomatic Medicine: theory, physiology, and practice*, vol. 2, monograph 2. International Universities Press, 1989, Madison CT.

Eisenberg DM, Delbanco TL, Berkey CS, Kaptchuk TJ, et al. Cognitive behavioral techniques for hypertension: are they effective? *Annals of Internal Medicine* 1993; 118:964–72.

FPN. Research is showing healthful effects of laughter. *Family Practice News* 1992; May 15:52a–52b.

Flach J, Seachrist L. Mind-body meld may boost immunity. *Journal of the National Cancer Institute* 1994; 86(4):256–58.

Friedman HS, VandenBos GR. Disease-prone and self-healing personalities. *Hospital and Community Psychiatry* 1992; 43(12):1177–79.

Gruber BL, Hersh SP, Hall NRS, et al. Immunological responses of breast cancer patients to behavioral interventions. *Biofeedback and Self-Regulation* 1993; 18(1):1–22.

Guthrie E, Creed F, Dawson D, Tomenson B. A controlled trial of psychological treatment for the irritable bowel syndrome. *Gastroenterology* 1991; 100:450–52.

House JS, Robbins C, Metzner HL. The association of social relationships and activities with mortality: prospective evidence from the Tecumseh community health study. *American Journal of Epidemiology* 1982; 116(1):123–40.

Karasek RA, Theorell T, Schwartz JE, et al. Job characteristics in relation to the prevalence of myocardial infarction in the US Health Examination Survey (HES) and the Health and Nutrition Examination Survey (HANES). *American Journal of Public Health* 1988; 78:910–18.

Kerkvliet GJ. Music therapy may help control cancer pain. *Journal of the National Cancer Institute* 1990; 82(5):350–52.

Kiecolt-Glaser JK and Glaser R. Psychological influences on immunity: implications for AIDS. *American Psychologist* 1988; 43(11):892–98.

Kiecolt-Glaser JK, Garner W, Speicher C, et al. Psychosocial modifiers of immunocompetence in medical students. *Psychosomatic Medicine* 1984; 46(1):7–41.

Kiecolt-Glaser JK, Marucha PT, Malarkey WB, et al. Slowing of wound healing by psychological stress. *Lancet* 1995; 346;1194–96.

Lown B, Desilva RA, Reich P, Murawski BJ. *American Journal of Psychiatry* 1980; 137(11):1325–35.

Marriott C, Harshbarger D. The hollow holiday: Christmas, a time of death in Appalachia. *Omega—Journal of Death and Dying* 1973 (Winter); 4(4):259–66.

Massing W, Angermeyer MC. Myocardial infarction on various days of the week. *Psychological Medicine* 1985; 15:851–57.

Phillips DP, Feldman KA. A dip in deaths before ceremonial occasions: some new relationships between social integration and mortality. *American Sociological Review* 1973; 38(6):678–96.

Phillips DP, Ruth TE, Wagner LM. Psychology and survival. *Lancet* 1993; 342:1142–45.

Rider MS, Achterberg J, Lawlis GF, et al. Effect of immune system imagery on secretory IgA. *Biofeedback and Self-Regulation* 1990; 15(4):317–33.

Rozanski A, Bairey N, Krantz DS, et al. Mental stress and the induction of silent myocardial ischemia in patients with coronary artery disease. *New England Journal of Medicine* 1988; 318:1005–12.

Schwartz SP, Taylor AE, Scharff L, Blanchard EB. Behaviorally treated irritable bowel syndrome patients: a four year follow-up. *Behavior Research and Therapy* 1990; 28(4):331–35.

Shaw G, Srivastava ED, Sadlier M, et al. Stress management for irritable bowel syndrome: a controlled trial. *Digestion* 1991; 50:36–42.

Shekelle RB, Gale M, Ostfeld AM, Oglesby P. Hostility, risk of coronary heart disease, and mortality. *Psychosomatic Medicine* 1983; 45(2):109–14.

Simonton OC, Matthews-Simonton S, Sparks TF. Psychological intervention in the treatment of cancer. *Psychosomatics* 1980; 21(3):226–33.

Spiegel D, Bloom JR. Group therapy and hypnosis reduce metastatic breast carcinoma pain. *Psychosomatic Medicine* 1983; 45(4):333–39.

Spiegel D, Kraemer HC, Bloom JR, Gottheil E. Effect of psychosocial treatment on survival of patients with metastatic breast cancer. *Lancet* 1989:888–91.

Taggart P, Carruthers M, Somerville W. Electrocardiogram, plasma catecholamines an lipids and their modification by oxyprenolol when speaking before an audience. *Lancet* 1973:341–46.

Taggart P, Gibbons D, Somerville W. Some effects of motor car driving on the normal and abnormal heart. *British Medical Journal* 1969; 4:130–34.

Thompson DR, Pohl JEF, Sutton TW. Acute myocardial infarction and day of the week. *American Journal of Cardiology* 1992; 69:266–67.

Vincent S, Thompson JH. The effects of music upon the human blood pressure. *Lancet* 1929:534–37.

Zimmerman LM, Pierson MA, Marker J. Effects of music on patient anxiety in coronary care units. *Heart Lung* 1988; 17:560–66.

Relaxation and meditation

Achterberg J, Kenner C, Casey D. Behavioral strategies for the reduction of pain and anxiety associated with orthopedic trauma. *Biofeedback and Self-Regulation* 1989; 14(2):101–14.

REFERENCES FOR RELAXATION AND MEDITATION CHAPTER

Bridge LR, Benson P, Pietroni PC, Priest RG. Relaxation and imagery in the treatment of breast cancer. *British Medical Journal* 1988; 297(5):1169–72.

Ceccio CM. Postoperative pain relief through relaxation in elderly patients with fractured hips. *Orthopaedic Nursing* 1984; 3(3):11–19.

Dahl J, Melin L, Brorson L-O, Schollin J. Effects of a broad-spectrum behavior modification treatment program on children with refractory epileptic seizures. *Epilepsia* 1985; 26(4):303–09.

Dahl J, Melin L, Lund L. Effects of a contingent relaxation treatment program on adults with refractory epileptic seizures. *Epilepsia* 1987; 28:125–32.

Deepak KK, Manchanda SK, Maheshwari MC. Meditation improves clinicoelectroencephalographic measures in drug-resistant epileptics. *Biofeedback and Self-regulation* 1994; 19(1):25–40.

Eppley KR, Abrams AI, Shear J. Differential effects of relaxation techniques on trait anxiety: a meta-analysis. *Journal of Clinical Psychology* 1989; 45:957–74.

Flaherty GG, Fitzpatrick JJ. Relaxation technique to increase comfort level of postoperative patients: a preliminary study. *Nursing Research* 1978; 27(6):352–55.

Holden-Lund C. Effects of relaxation with guided imagery on surgical stress and wound healing. *Research in Nursing and Health* 1988; 11:235–44.

Kabat-Zinn J, Lipworth L, Burney R, Sellers W. Four year follow-up of a meditation-based program for the self-regulation of chronic pain: treatment outcomes and compliance. *Clinical Journal of Pain* 1986; 2:159–73.

Kabat-Zinn J, Massion AO, Kristeller J, et al. Effectiveness of a meditation-based stress reduction program in the treatment of anxiety disorders. *American Journal of Psychiatry* 1992; 149(7):936–43.

Kiecolt-Glaser JK, Glaser R, Williger D, et al. Psychosocial enhancement of immunocompetence in a geriatric population. *Health Psychology* 1985; 4(1):25–41.

Lawlis GF, Selby D, Hinnant D, McCoy CE. Reduction of postoperative pain parameters by presurgical relaxation instructions for spinal pain patients. *Spine* 1985; 10(7):649–51.

Lazarus AA. Psychiatric problems precipitated by transcendental meditation. *Psychological Reports* 1975; 10:39–74.

Miller JJ, Fletcher K, Kabat-Zinn J. Three year follow-up and clinical implications of a mindfulness meditation-based stress reduction intervention in the treatment of anxiety disorders. *General Hospital Psychiatry* 1995; 17:192–200.

Orme-Johnson D. Medical care utilization and the transcendental meditation program. *Psychosomatic Medicine* 1987; 49:493–507.

Puskarich CA, Whitman S, Dell J, et al. Controlled examination of effects of progressive relaxation training on seizure reduction. *Epilepsia* 1992; 33(4):675–80.

Rousseau A, Hermann BP, Whitman S. Effects of progressive relaxation on epilepsy: analysis of a series of cases. *Psychological Reports* 1985; 57:1203–12.

Shapiro DH. Adverse effects of meditation: a preliminary investigation of long-term meditators. *International Journal of Psychosomatics* 1992; 39:62–67.

Smith JC. Psychotherapeutic effects of transcendental meditation with controls for expectation of relief and daily sitting. *Journal of Consulting and Clinical Psychology* 1976; 44(4):630–37.

Stuckey SJ, Jacobs A, Goldfarb J. EMG biofeedback training, relaxation training, and placebo for the relief of chronic back pain. *Perceptual and Motor Skills* 1986; 63:1023–36.

Wallace RK, Silver J, Mills PJ, et al. Systolic blood pressure and long-term practice of the Transcendental Meditation and TM-Sidhi program: effects of TM on systolic blood pressure. *Psychosomatic Medicine* 1983; 45(1):41–46.

Walsh R, Rauche L. The precipitation of acute psychoses by intensive meditation in individuals with a history of schizophrenia. *American Journal of Psychiatry* 1979; 138(8):185–86.

Whitman S, Dell J, Legion V, et al. Progressive relaxation for seizure reduction. *Journal of Epilepsy* 1990; 3:17–22.

Spiritual healing

Benor DJ. *Healing Research: Holistic Energy Medicine and Spirituality, Volume 1.* Helix Editions, 1993, United Kingdom.

Benor DJ. Survey of spiritual healing research. *Complementary Medical Research* 1990; 4(30):9–33.

Beutler JJ, Attevelt JTM, Schouten SA, et al. Paranormal healing and hypertension. *British Medical Journal* 1988; 296:1491–94.

Byrd RC. Positive therapeutic effects of intercessory prayer in a coronary care unit population. *Southern Medical Journal* 1988; 81:826–29.

Collipp PJ. The efficacy of prayer: a triple-blind study. *Medical Times* 1969; 97:201–04.

Galton F. Statistical inquiries into the efficacy of prayer. *Fortnightly Review* 1872; 12:125–35. Excerpted in "Does prayer preserve?" by CG Roland, in *Archives of Internal Medicine* 1970; 125:580–87.

Joyce CRB, Welldon RMC. The objective efficacy of prayer: a double-blind clinical trial. *Journal of Chronic Disease* 1965; 18:367–77.

Koss JD. Expectations and outcomes for patients given mental health care or spiritist healing in Puerto Rico. *American Journal of Psychiatry* 1987; 144:56–61.

Levin JS, Vanderpool HY. Is frequent religious attendance really conducive to better health?: toward an epidemiology of religion. *Social Science and Medicine* 1987; 24(7):589–600.

Miscellaneous therapies

Aaron RK, Ciomber DM. Therapeutic effects of electromagnetic fields in the stimulation of connective tissue repair. *Journal of Cellular Biochemistry* 1993; 52(1):42–46.

Abraham M, Devi NS, Sheela R. Inhibiting effect of jasmine flowers on lactation. *Indian Journal of Medical Research* 1979; 69:88–92.

Baron RA. Environmentally-induced positive effect:Its impact on self-efficacy, task performance, negotiation, and conflict. *Journal of Applied Social Psychology* 1990; 20:368–84.

Barrett-Connor E, Khaw K-T. Absence of an inverse relation of dehydroepiandrosterone sulfate with cardiovascular disease mortality in postmenopausal women. *New England Journal of Medicine* 1987; 317:711.

Barrett-Connor E, Khaw K-T, Yen SSC. A prospective study of dehydroepiandrosterone sulfate, mortality and cardiovascular disease. *New England Journal of Medicine* 1986; 315:1519–24.

Bassett CAL. Beneficial effects of electromagnetic fields. *Journal of Cellular Biochemistry* 1993; 51:387–93.

Bassett IB, Pannowitz DL, Barnetson RSC. A comparative study of tea-tree oil versus benzoylperoxide in the treatment of acne. *Medical Journal of Australia* 1990; 153:455–58.

Bell GD, Doran J. Gallstone dissolution in man using an essential oil preparation. *British Medical Journal* 1979; i:24.

Bocci V, Paulesu L. Studies on the biological effects of ozone:1. Induction of interferon gamma on human leukocytes. *Haemalogica* 1990; 75:510–15.

Brackowski R, Zubelewicz B, Romanowski W, et al. Preliminary study on modulation of the biological effect of tumor necrosis factor alpha in advanced cancer patients by the pineal gland melatonin. *Journal of Biological Regulators and Homeostatic Agents* 1994; 8(3):77–80.

Brown DD, Mucci WG, Hetzler RK, Knowlton RG. Cardiovascular and ventilatory responses during formalized T'ai Chi Chuan exercise. *Research Quarterly for Exercise and Sport* 1989; 60:246–50.

Buck, DS, Nidorf DM, Addino JG. Comparison of two topical preparations for the treatment of onychomycosis: Melaleuca Alternifolia (tea tree) oil and clotrimazole. *Journal of Family Practice* 1994; 38(6):601–05.

Capanna R, Donati D, Masetti C, et al. Effect of electromagnetic fields on patients undergoing massive bone graft following bone tumor resection. *Clinical Orthopaedics and Related Research* 1994; 306:213–21.

Cassileth BR, Lusk EJ, Guerry D, et al. Survival and quality of life among patients receiving unproven as compared with conventional cancer therapy. *New England Journal of Medicine* 1991; 324:1180–85.

Creagan ET, Moertel CG, O'Fallon JR, et al. Failure of high-dose vitamin C (ascorbic acid) therapy to benefit patients with advanced cancer:a controlled trial. *New England Journal of Medicine* 1979; 301:687–90.

Dale A, Cornwell S. The role of lavender oil in relieving perineal discomfort following childbirth: a blind randomized clinical trial. *Journal of Advanced Nursing* 1994; 19:89–96.

Dew MJ, Evans BK, Rhodes J. Peppermint oil for the irritable bowel syndrome: a multicentre trial. *British Journal of Clinical Practice* 1984; 38:394–98.

Ebeling P, Kolvisto VA. Physiological importance of dehydroepiandrosterone. *Lancet* 1994; 343:1479–81.

Ekman AC, Leppaluoto J, Huttunen P, et al. Ethanol inhibits melatonin secretion in healthy volunteers in a dose-dependent randomized double-blind cross-over study. *Journal of Clinical Endocrinology and Metabolism* 1993; 77(3):780–83.

Ellis WR, Bell GD. Treatment of biliary duct stones with a terpene preparation. *British Medical Journal* 1981; 282:611.

Ellis WR, Sommerville KW, Whitten BH, Bell GD. Pilot study of combination treatment for gallstones with medium dose chenodeoxycholic acid and a terpene preparation. *British Medical Journal* 1984; 289:153–56.

Elson CE, Underbakke GL, Hanson P, et al. Impact of lemongrass oil, an essential oil, on serum cholesterol. *Lipids* 1989; 24(8):677–79.

Folkard S, Arendt J, Clark M. Can melatonin improve shift workers' tolerance of the night shift? Some preliminary findings. *Chronobiology International* 1993; 10(5):315–20.

Garfinkel D, Laudon M, Nof D, Zisapel N. Improvement of sleep quality in elderly people by controlled-release melatonin. *Lancet* 1995; 346:541–44.

Gobel H, Schmidt G, Soyka D. Effect of peppermint and eucalyptus oil preparations on neurophysiological and experimental algesimetric headache parameters. *Cephalalgia* 1994; 14:228–34.

Gordon GB, Bush TL, Helzsouer KJ, et al. Relationship of serum levels of dehydroepiandrosterone sulfate to the risk of developing postmenopausal breast cancer. *Cancer Research* 1990; 50:3859–62.

Grier MT, Meyers DG. So much writing, so little science: a review of 37 years of literature on edetate sodium chelation therapy. *Annals of Pharmacotherapy* 1993; 27:1504–09.

Guldager B, Jelnes R, Jorgensen SJ, et al. EDTA treatment of intermittent claudication—a double-blind, placebo-controlled study. *Journal of Internal Medicine* 1992; 231:261–67.

Huether G. The contribution of extrapineal sites of melatonin synthesis to circulating melatonin levels in higher vertebrates. *Experientia* 1993; 49(8):665–70.

Jacobs MR, Hornfeldt CS. Melaleuca oil poisoning. *Clinical Toxicology* 1994; 32(4):461–64.

Jin P. Efficacy of T'ai Chi, brisk walking, meditation, and reading in reducing mental and emotional stress. *Journal of Psychosomatic Research* 1992; 36(4):361–70.

229

Kirk-Smith, MD, Van Toller C, Dodd DH. Unconscious odour conditioning in human subjects. *Biological Psychology* 1983; 17:221–31.

Knasko SC. Ambient odor's effect on creativity, mood, and perceived health. *Chemical Senses* 1992; 17(1):27–35.

Knasko SC. Performance, mood, and health during exposure to intermittent odors. *Archives of Environmental Health* 1993; 48(5):305–08.

Leuschner M, Leuschner U, Lazarovici D, et al. Dissolution of gallstones with an ursodeoxycholic acid menthol preparation: a controlled prospective double blind trial. *Gut* 1988; 29:428–32.

Lissoni P, Barni S, Ardizzoia A, et al. *Cancer* 1994; 73(3):699–701.

Ludvigson HW, Rottman TR. Effects of ambient odors of lavender and cloves on cognition, memory, affect and mood. *Chemical Senses* 1989; 14(4):525–36.

Mammi GI, Rocchi R, Cadossi R, et al. The electrical stimulation of tibial osteotomies. *Clinical Orthopaedics and Related Research* 1993; 288:246–53.

Mehlman MA, Borek C. Toxicity and biochemical mechanisms of ozone. *Environmental Research* 1987; 42:36–53.

Mitchell LE, Sprecher DL, Borecki IB, et al. Evidence for an association between dehydroepiandrosterone sulfate and nonfatal, premature myocardial infarction in males. *Circulation* 1994; 89:89–93.

Nash P, Gould SR, Barnardo DE. Peppermint oil does not relieve the pain of irritable bowel syndrome. *British Journal of Clinical Practice* 1986; 40:292–93.

Paulesu L, Luzzi E, Bocci V. Studies on the biological effects of ozone: 2. Induction of tumor necrosis factor (TNF-a) on human leukocytes. *Lymphokine and Cytokine Research* 1991; 10(5):409–12.

Pennington GM, Danley DL, Sumko MH, et al. Pulsed, non-thermal, high frequency electromagnetic energy (DIAPULSE) in the treatment of grade I and grade II ankle sprains. *Military Medicine* 1993; 158(2):101–04.

Petrie K, Dawson AG, Thompson L, Brook R. A double-blind trial of melatonin as a treatment for jet lag in international cabin crew. *Biological Psychiatry* 1993; 33(7):526–30.

Rees WDW, Evans BK, Rhodes J. Treating irritable bowel syndrome with peppermint oil. *British Medical Journal* 1979; 2:835–36.

Regelson W, Loria R, Kalimi M. Dehydroepiandrosterone (DHEA)—the "mother steroid." *Annals of the New York Academy of Sciences* 1994; 719:553–63.

Rose JE, Behm FM. Inhalation of vapor from black pepper extract reduces smoking withdrawal symptoms. *Drug and Alcohol Dependence* 1994; 34:225–29.

Rybeck CH, Swenson R. The effect of oral administration of refined sugar on muscle strength. *Journal of Manipulative and Physiological Therapeutics* 1980; 3(3):155–61.

Salzberg CA, Cooper-Vastola SA, Perez F, et al. The effects of non-thermal pulsed electromagnetic energy on wound healing of pressure ulcers in spinal cord-injured patients: a randomized, double-blind study. *Ostomy/Wound Management* 1995; 41(3):42–48.

Shrivastav P, George K, Balasubramaniam N, et al. Suppression of puerperal lactation using jasmine flowers (Jasminum sambac). *Australia and New Zealand Journal of Obstetrics and Gynecology* 1988; 28:68–71.

Sisken BF, Walker J, Orgel M. Prospects on clinical applications of electrical stimulation for nerve regeneration. *Journal of Cellular Biochemistry* 1993; 51(4):404–09.

Sommerville KW, Ellis WR, Whitten BH, et al. Stones in the common bile duct: experience with medical dissolution therapy. *Postgraduate Medical Journal* 1985; 61:313–16.

Stevenson C. The psychophysiological effects of aromatherapy massage following cardiac surgery. *Complementary Therapies in Medicine* 1994; 2(1):27–35.

230

Sullivan JB, Rumack BH, Thomas H, et al. Pennyroyal oil poisoning and hepatotoxicity. *Journal of the American Medical Association* 1979; 242(26):2873–74.

Sweet F, Kao M-S, Lee S-CD, et al. Ozone selectively inhibits growth of human cancer cells. *Science* 1980; 209:931–32.

Triano JJ. Muscle strength testing as a diagnostic screen for supplemental nutrition therapy: a blind study. *Journal of Manipulative and Physiological Therapeutics* 1982; 5(4):179–82.

Tse S-K, Bailey DM. T'ai Chi and postural control in the well elderly. *American Journal of Occupational Therapy* 1992; 46(4):295–300.

Vallance WB. Pennyroyal poisoning: a fatal case. *Lancet* 1955; 2:850–51.

van Rij AM, Solomon C, Packer SGK, Hopkins WG. Chelation therapy for intermittent claudication: a double-blind, randomized, controlled trial. *Circulation* 1994; 90:1194–99.

van Vollenhoven RF, Engleman EG, Mcguire JL. An open study of dehydroepiandrosterone in systemic lupus erythematosus. *Arthritis and Rheumatism* 1994; 9:1305–10.

Vickers AJ. *Massage and Aromatherapy: a guide for health professionals.* Chapman and Hall, 1996, London.

Vodovnik L, Karba R. Treatment of chronic wounds by means of electric and electromagnetic fields. *Medical and Biological Engineering and Computing* 1992; 30:257–66.

Warm JS, Dember WM, Parasuraman R. Effects of fragrances on vigilance performance and stress. *Perfumer & Flavorist* 1990; 15(15):17–18.

Webb NJ, Pitt WR. Eucalyptus oil poisoning in childhood: 41 cases in south-east Queensland. *Journal of Paediatrics and Child Health* 1993; 29:368–371.

Wells KH, Latino J, Gavalchin J, Poiesz BJ. Inactivation of human immunodeficiency virus type 1 by ozone in vitro. *Blood* 1991; 78(7):1882–90.

Wilkinson S. Aromatherapy and massage in palliative care. *International Journal of Palliative Nursing* 1995; 1(1):21–30.

Wisniewski TL, Hilton CW, Morse EV, Svec F. The relationship of serum DHEA-S and cortisol levels to measures of immune function in human immunodeficiency virus-related illness. *American Journal of Medical Science* 1993; 305(2):79–83.

Zumoff B, Levin J, Rosenfeld RS, et al. Abnormal 24-hr mean plasma concentrations of dehydroepiandrosterone and dehydroepiandrosterone sulfate in women with primary operable breast cancer. *Cancer Research* 1981; 41:3360–63.

INDEX

ACKNOWLEDGEMENTS

First and foremost, my thanks to Arthur Naiman. No paternity test needed—this book is as much his as it is mine. It was his idea, and his meticulous editing vastly improved the end product. Arthur went above and beyond the duties of a publisher, editor, fellow writer and friend. It was a joy getting to know his generous spirit and sarcastic wit, and I thank him from the bottom of my heart.

The other person to whom I owe most for this book is my dear friend Charlea Massion MD, who excels at many things but perhaps most at the art of living. Charlea provided me a Santa Cruz writing haven (replete with sunny rooms, roses and poppies, strictly enforced walks on the beach, great produce and host cats Max, Chiara and Quince). Without Charlea's sanity, friendship, multi-faceted support and deadpan humor, this book would have taken years longer.

I'd also like to thank the feminists-yearning-for-our-past-lives-in-collectives group, especially Thea Lee, Vickie Leonard, Cindy Pearson, Fran Pollner and Stella Dawson—our feasts, conversations and especially our laughter are life-sustaining;

Ted Kaptchuk OMD, for inspiration, unwavering support, arcane historical details and always saying just the right thing at times of crisis;

my brother Stu, sister-in-law Eileen, nephew Danny, niece Pam and especially my mother, Aline Fugh Berman, for tolerating crabbiness and neglect during this process (and for supplying many meals);

Ben Perez JD, for love, support and thousands of wonderful meals, and for putting up with me for all those years;

Quing Wu OMD, for always expanding the boundaries of what is possible;

Harry Coulter PhD, who reviewed the homeopathy chapter and delivered blini and caviar, among other fine meals;

Mark Blumenthal, for his enthusiasm, generous nature, modesty and a careful reading of the herbs chapter;

Pam Stratton MD, who brought me lunch for two months during a bad patch;

the fabulous librarians and interlibrary loan folks at the NIH library and the George Washington University Medical School library;

Bruce Stadel MD, for invaluable help with the clinical trials chapter;

Marc Micozzi MD PhD, for scintillating conversations;

Jamie McGregor MD, for enthusiasm and wonderful photography;

John McPartland DO, who clarified points on manipulative therapies (and who always improves my state of mind);

Andrew Vickers, who kindly shared the manuscript of his aromatherapy book with me;

Michael Balick PhD, for many helpful comments and for FedExing books on an emergency basis;

Susan McCallister, whose attention to detail improved the book tremendously;

David Freeman, for coming up with the title;

Lane Baldwin and Dat Lam at Computer Care, who stayed late on a Saturday to rescue data from a recalcitrant computer;

those without whom I wouldn't have survived medical training—especially Danny Lawlor MD, Jane Dalglish Willis MD, John Jewett MD, Meg Rosenberg MD, Kenneth Hill MD, Lee Olson MD, Meggie Byrne MD, Taffy Dorsey MD, Joy Williams, Jim Lewis MD, John Harmon MD, Jim Calvert MD and Arthur Hoyte MD;

the National Institutes of Health Minority Access to Research Careers program;

and my teachers at the University of the District of Columbia, who inspired me to be a scientist—especially Robert Martin PhD, Norman Kondo PhD, Marian Johnson-Thompson PhD, Caroline Cousin PhD and Edward Rogers PhD.

For various kindnesses during this project, I thank Nancy J. Alexander PhD, Rocio Aragon DC, Bev Baker, Damaris Christiansen, Felipe Chirinos, Carolyn Clancy MD, Katie Clark, Devra Lee Davis PhD, Bobbie Diester PhD, Brian Dressler MD, Roger Edwards PhD, Daniel Eskinazi DDS PhD, Freddie Ann Hoffman MD, Alan Gaby MD, Herman J. Glass DC, Jim Gordon MD, Steve Groft PhD, Dick Grossman, Florence Haseltine MD PhD, Michael Hennessey, Chris Henry MD, Joe Jacobs MD, Steve Kaufman MD, Joe Kelaghan MD, Fredi Kronenberg PhD, Floyd Leaders PhD, David de Leeuw, Luke McBride, Rob McCaleb, Fitzhugh Mullan MD, Helen Rodriguez-Trias MD, Isidore Rosmarin, Tina Pirrone, J.P. Smith, Peter Thibodeau DC, Alan Trachtenberg MD, Michael Wallis, Jackie Wootton and Roo.